Computerised Axial Tomography in Oncology

European Seminar on Computerised Axial Tomography in Clinical Practice (2nd :1980 : London, England)

Computerised Axial Tomography in Oncology

Edited by

JANET E. HUSBAND

and

PAULINE A. HOBDAY

Royal Marsden Hospital and Institute of Cancer
Research, Sutton, Surrey

CHURCHILL LIVINGSTONE
EDINBURGH LONDON MELBOURNE AND NEW YORK 1981

CHURCHILL LIVINGSTONE
Medical Division of Longman Group Limited

Distributed in the United States of America by
Churchill Livingstone Inc., 19 West 44th Street, New York,
N.Y. 10036, and by associated companies,
branches and representatives throughout
the world.

First published 1981

ISBN 0 443 02196 1

British Library Cataloguing in Publication Data
Computerised axial tomography in oncology.
   1. Cancer – Research – Congresses
   2. Tomography – Data processing – Congresses
   I. Husband, Janet E.   II. Hobday, Pauline A.
   616.99 2 0072   RC267   80-42228

Printed and bound in Great Britain by
William Clowes (Beccles) Limited, Beccles and London

Preface

Following the successful European Seminar on Computerised Axial Tomography in Clinical Practice held in London during October 1976, a second Seminar was held on computed Tomography in Oncology in London in February 1980, under the patronage of the Duke of Devonshire MC PC, Chairman of the Cancer Research Campaign.

ESCAT 2 was organised because there is a growing need to define the role of whole body CT scanning in the management of patients with malignant disease. Information is now available regarding the diagnostic capability of CT but its practical value in the staging of specific tumours, monitoring therapeutic response and in radiotherapy treatment planning has not yet been fully evaluated.

This symposium presented a critical assessment of CT in oncology and stimulated much discussion. It is hoped that the interchange of ideas has helped to draw up guidelines so that CT may be used as effectively as possible in the detection and treatment of cancer.

Sutton, 1981

J.S. Macdonald
Janet E. Husband
Pauline Hobday

Acknowledgements

The Chairman and Committee of ESCAT 2 greatly acknowledge the contribution and assistance of all those who helped to organise this Conference. These include Mr Christopher Hicks and Mrs Helen McLoughlin of EMI Medical Ltd who handled much of the organisation and hotel arrangements and EMI Medical Ltd for all their financial assistance. We would also like to thank Miss Patricia Gilbe, Mrs Janice O'Donnell and Mrs Rosemary Sewell for their invaluable work.

The Organising Committee would like to take this opportunity of acknowledging the generosity and support given to the CT Scanning Unit at the Royal Marsden Hospital by the Cancer Research Campaign and the Department of Health and Social Security.

Organising Committee

Chairman: Dr J.S. MACDONALD

Secretaries: Dr JANET HUSBAND
Mrs PAULINE HOBDAY

Members: Dr N.J. HODSON
Dr R.P. PARKER
Dr C.A. PARSONS

Contributors

Professor R.J. Berry,
Department of Oncology and Physics as Applied to Medicine, Middlesex Hospital Medical School, London

Professor Jonathan Best,
Department of Medical Radiology, University of Edinburgh, Scotland

Dr George Blackledge, C.R.C.,
Department of Medical Oncology, University of Manchester, Manchester

Dr A. Bridier,
Physics Department, Institut Gustave Roussy, 94800 Villejuif, France

Mr K.J. Cassell,
Royal Marsden Hospital, Sutton, Surrey

Dr Claus Claussen,
Department of Radiology, Freie Universitat Berlin, Klinikum Charlottenburg and Steglitz, Berlin-West, Germany

Dr J.R. Cunningham,
The Ontario Cancer Institute, Toronto, Canada

Dr J. Doucette,
Massachusetts General Hospital, Boston, Massachusetts 02114, U.S.A.

Dr A. Dutreix,
Physics Department, Institut Gustave Roussy, 94800 Villejuif, France

Dr W.A. Fuchs,
Department of Diagnostic Radiology, University Hospital, Bern, Switzerland

Dr M. Haertel,
Department of Diagnostic Radiology, University Hospital, Bern Switzerland

Mrs Pauline Hobday,
Physics Department, Royal Marsden Hospital, Sutton, Surrey

Dr N.J. Hodson,
Royal Sussex County Hospital, Brighton, Sussex

Dr J.E. Husband,
Royal Marsden Hospital, Sutton, Surrey

Professor I Isherwood,
Department of Diagnostic Radiology, University of Manchester, Manchester

Ms Wendy Julian,
Department of Oncology and Physics as Applied to Medicine, Middlesex Hospital Medical School, London

Dr I. Kelsey Fry,
St Bartholomew's Hospital, West Smithfield, London EC1

Dr I-L Lamm,
Department of Oncology and Radiation Physics, University Hospital, S-221 85 Lund, Sweden

Dr T.G. Landberg,
Department of Oncology and Radiation Physics, University Hospital, S-221 85 Lund, Sweden

Dr M.O. Leach,
Physics Department, Royal Marsden Hospital, Sutton, Surrey

Dr J.S. Macdonald,
Department of Radiology, Royal Marsden Hospital, Sutton, Surrey

Dr T.R. Moller,
Department of Oncology and Radiation Physics, University Hospital, S-221 85 Lund, Sweden

Dr J.E. Munzenrider,
Massachusetts General Hospital, Boston, Massachusetts 02114, U.S.A.

Dr N. Noscoe,
Department of Oncology and Physics as Applied to Medicine, Middlesex Hospital Medical School, London

Dr R.P. Parker,
Physics Department, Royal Marsden Hospital, Sutton, Surrey

Dr C. Parsons,
Royal Marsden Hospital, Sutton, Surrey

Professor M.J. Peckham,
Department of Radiotherapy and Oncology, Royal Marsden Hospital, Sutton, Surrey

Dr K. Damgaard-Pedersen,
Department of Diagnostic Radiology, Rigshospitalet, University of Copenhagen, Denmark

Dr M. Pfister,
Research Fellow, German Hospital, Duenos Aires, Argentina

Professor B.R. Pullan,
Department of Medical Biophysics, University of Manchester, Manchester

Dr R.T. Ritchings,
Department of Computation, University of Manchester Institute of Science and Technology, Manchester

Mr J. Twydle,
Department of Oncology and Physics as Applied to Medicine, Middlesex Hospital Medical School, London

Dr J. Van Dyk,
The Ontario Cancer Institute, Toronto, Canada

Dr L. Verhey,
Massachusetts General Hospital, Boston, Massachusetts 02114, U.S.A.

Dr P. Vock,
Department of Diagnostic Radiology, University Hospital, Bern, Switzerland

Dr S. Webb,
Physics Department, Royal Marsden Hospital, Sutton, Surrey

Dr Otto H. Wegner,
Department of Radiology, Freie Universitat Berlin, Klinikum Charlottenburg and Steglitz, Berlin-West, Germany

Contents

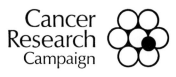

(British Empire Cancer Campaign for Research)

Cancer Research Campaign
2 Carlton House Terrace, London SW1Y 5AR
01-930 8972

4 February 1980

INTRODUCTION

It is a pleasure to welcome you to London and to ESCAT 2. It is apt that a European Seminar on Computed Tomography in Oncology should be held at this time.

Cancer is one of the most serious health problems which faces us at present with 1.4 million deaths in Europe each year.

The first whole body CT scanner was announced only four years ago but now these are being installed in increasing numbers throughout Europe. It is right that those concerned with oncology and with the application of this great advance in imaging should pause, learn from each other and think together about the application of this new and sensitive technology which has such relevance to the cancer problem.

The Duke of Devonshire MC PC
Chairman of the Cancer Research Campaign

1. Computed tomography in a clinical setting

J. S. MACDONALD

CT of the brain is well established and well documented and there is no argument about its place in neuroradiology nor about its cost effectiveness in the management of these patients. The position as regards the general purpose of the whole body scanner is different; there is argument about what it can do, where it should be sited, what size of population it should serve and whether or not it costs too much.

It was decided to hold a symposium devoted to CT in oncology because, whatever place CT eventually finds in the wider realm of diagnostic radiology, its place in the whole management of certain cancer patients would appear to be considerable, ranging from primary diagnosis in the form of needle aspiration for definitive histology, through staging and assessing the volume of tumour present, to the more accurate delineation of the volume to be irradiated. Then there is the assessment of the response of tumours to treatment and the delineation of residual disease if any.

The timing of this symposium was apt and to quote His Grace The Duke of Devonshire, Patron of ESCAT 2:

> The first whole body CT scanner was announced only four years ago, but now they are being installed in increasing numbers throughout Europe. It is right that those concerned with oncology and with the application of this great advance in imaging should pause, learn from each other and think together about the use of this new and sensitive technology which has such relevance to the cancer problem.

Discussion on CT in oncology is particularly useful at this time so that thought can feed on ideas developed during the initial enthusiasm generated by the installation of these machines and particularly when the new generation of scanners is arriving on the scene. There is enthusiastic talk about scannograms, thinner cuts, faster times, angled gantries and new table movements. These are considerable and useful advances but they must be used logically and in the proper way to push forward knowledge. We have been here before in standard tomography when the multidirectional machines were introduced and innumerable thinner and thinner slices were taken in inappropriate places when a thicker slice at a slightly different level would have given as much information. The new generation of scanners should be welcomed. They should teach us a great deal, but let us build on what is already known and beware of being too hasty.

The new facilities will allow further study of the behaviour of tumours particularly under treatment and the way in which they handle contrast media. Subsequent chapters will describe how far physics has progressed and it will be up to the clinicians to use this information.

It is my brief to take a broad view of CT in oncology. The facts and figures of individual research will follow but the size of the problem must not be underrated. There are 1.4 million deaths from cancer in Europe each year; 3 out of 10 people will contract cancer at some time in their life and 2 out of these 3 will die of it. That is the size of the oncologist's problem (Ennals, 1978).

Cancer affects every system and all parts of the body and there is not much time to deal with it in the clinical phase. Even when active tumour growth has been induced, it takes time for a clinically demonstrated mass to appear. Tumours do not grow regularly, parts advance while others necrose, their rate of enlargement follows no simple law but there is, nevertheless, some relevance in statements such as that of Collins, Loeffler & Tivey (1956). The first 20 doublings in the life of a cancer produce a minimal detectable lesion 1 mm in diameter. The second 20 doublings increase the bulk to 1 kilogram of tumour tissue and bring the patient close to the termination of the disease. It is difficult to get accurate histories about the time when tumours were first noticed and even harder to find measurements of precise size on which to base an assessment of growth rate (Smithers, 1960). The precision of the scanner in defining tumours is now able to help further along this road.

The treatment of patients with cancer is most effective when tumour bulk is small and localised or when the primary has been dealt with and deposits are discovered when small. The identification of tumours and deposits when still as small as possible has always been one of the aims of the diagnostic radiologist.

The scanner is the most sensitive means yet devised for using X-rays diagnostically; Under the most favourable conditions, such as the periphery of the lungs, deposits of only a few millimetres in diameter can be shown. It can show deposits in other parts of the lung, the mediastinum, the retrocrural area and the mesentery, more clearly and with greater confidence than any other available technique. For the first time the pancreas can be shown consistently. The scanner will define accurately the size of a deposit after it has burst out of the confines of a lymph node and can show the size of an associated soft tissue mass in what appears to be a relatively circumscribed tumour of bone.

There is now sufficient experience of general purpose CT scanners to see their place in the overall clinical setting of oncology and to apply their unique advantages to defining the precise location of some tumours, the extent of spread and their behaviour under treatment. It is imperative that this valuable imaging technique should not be wasted on areas where the information derived from the scanner will not change management of that particular patient nor further our knowledge of individual tumours. The sensitivity of the scanner in the lungs, the mediastinum and retroperitoneum has already improved staging in these areas, but specific questions have to be asked about each individual type of tumour as well as each anatomical region for meaningful answers to be forthcoming. The right questions can only be derived from the mass of information already known about the natural history of each tumour and its preferred mode of spread. There is no such thing as a cancer problem, but rather the problem of many types of cancer.

Much has been done with the scanner, but it has its weak points and failings too. It is not a piece of esoteric wizardry, the answer to all oncologists' prayers. It is another piece of diagnostic equipment to be used well. Scanning experience with the early machines has been disappointing, on the whole, in areas of the pelvis and the liver. Such areas must be identified and efforts must be concentrated on perfecting techniques to improve the quality of information, or find something else that will. It is in these situations that thinner cuts, faster scanning times, tilting gantries and new contrast techniques will help.

There is argument about the size of population that a general purpose CT scanner should serve. This is a big topic and not for discussion here, but when considering CT in oncology, it is reasonable that any centre large enough for example to support two megavoltage treatment machines, 4 radiotherapists or 1500 new patients per year, should have access to a scanner. There is argument, too, about where the scanner should be sited. The CT scanner is a piece of diagnostic equipment and it should therefore be sited in the diagnostic X-ray department.

It cannot be emphasised too strongly, however, that certainly in the climate of oncology, in order to get the best results from the scanner and the optimum benefit to the patients, there must be the very closest co-operation between diagnostic radiologists, radiotherapists, oncologists, physicists, radiographers both diagnostic and therapeutic and the physics staff. This co-operation is essential and there must be a real will to co-operate because of the inevitable stresses in an overworked department. These stresses will remain because in Europe in the foreseeable future there is little prospect of an adequate number of general purpose scanners to carry the service load, quite apart from any research. The load is constantly increasing because from the very nature of this sort of work 30 per cent are repeat scans and naturally the problem is complicated further if a scanner is serving more than one hospital or, for instance, if the treatment planning is being undertaken at a hospital remote from the scanner.

This leads on to the place of the CT scanner in radiotherapy treatment planning. A lot of work has been done on this and it would seem that it has an important role where curative radiotherapy, not merely palliation, is being planned (Macdonald et al, 1977; Husband et al, 1978; Hobday et al, 1979). Most radiotherapy treatment plans are built up on cross-sectional representations of the body at the level of the tumour and it has long been obvious that a true radiological cross section of the body at the level of the tumour would have many advantages.

In 1937 William Watson invented an apparatus for transverse axial tomography (Fig. 1.1) but because of all the problems caused by the Second World War very little was done about it. After the war, the apparatus was installed in the diagnostic X-ray department at the Royal Marsden Hospital in London (The Royal Cancer Hospital as it was then) where the first clinical transverse axial tomographs were taken (Stevenson, 1950). The quality of the radiographs taken by the prototype was very good as can be seen by referring to the original paper but, although interesting, they gave little extra diagnostic information. It was not used for treatment planning although its potential was recognised and it was abandoned. Subsequently, several commercial firms put transverse axial tomographs in the market and when the Royal Marsden Hospital in Surrey was built in 1962 one of these was installed in order to reassess its diagnostic potential and also to use it in conjunction with the newly designed treatment planning simulator.

The diagnostic application was found to be limited and only in two areas did the technique give information not otherwise readily shown on plain films and conven-

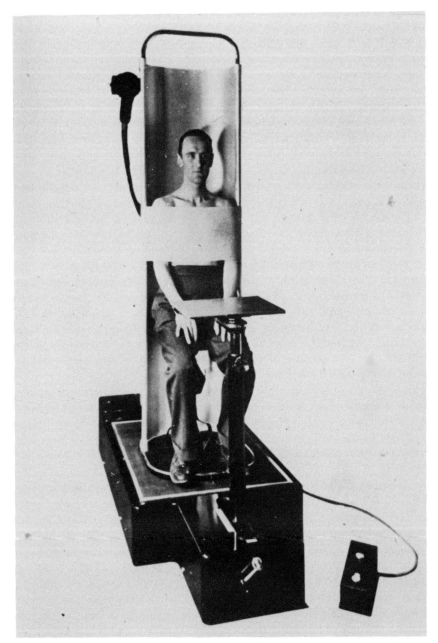

Fig. 1.1 William Watson's apparatus for transverse axial tomography. (Illustration given to the author by William Watson.)

tional tomography. These were enlarged nodes behind the manubrium of the sternum (Fig. 1.2) and enlarged subcarinal nodes which extended posteriorly without splaying the carina. Incidentally, these are two areas where CT has been

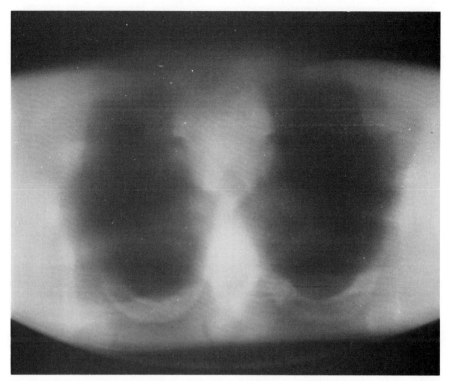

Fig. 1.2 Transverse axial tomograph of the thorax in a patient with Hodgkin's disease. There are enlarged anterior mediastinal nodes.

found to be particularly useful, confirming the early findings. A lot of work was done in the chest on treatment planning, mostly by A.J. Stacey, and although quite a few lessons were learned and these helped to improve treatment planning, this project was defeated by the lack of accurate end points because of the inherent blur (Figs. 1.2 and 1.3) of the tomographs and the all important fact that the treatment planning position could not be simulated because the patient had to sit erect in rather a constrained position while being rotated through 360 degrees. (Macdonald, 1964)

Transverse axial tomography produced adequate radiographs in the head and neck (Fig. 1.4) and thorax, but was disappointing below the diaphragm even with the introduction of contrast medium either by intravenous injection or retro-peritoneal insufflation.

To aid radiotherapy treatment planning, the outlines of the body, the tumour mass and the important structures were traced from the transverse axial tomograph, reduced to actual size and then the treatment plan was produced (Fig. 1.5).

Later Takahashi developed a transverse axial tomography apparatus which overcame the positioning problem by taking tomograms with the patient lying flat, but we never installed one of these machines as we had certain doubts about the accuracy of end points and the amount of further information which could be gleaned.

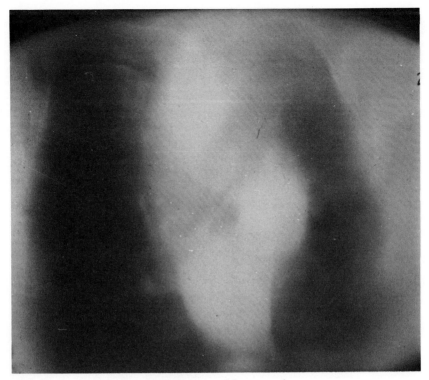

Fig. 1.3 Carcinoma of the bronchus, transverse axial tomograph.

As mentioned above, it is important to have the knowledge to know the right questions to ask in order to have a chance of getting the right answers. After a great deal of thought and work, it was found that phantoms could be planned very accurately, but it was different with patients. (Parker, 1979)

The right questions were being asked, but the technology was not available, and it needed the genius of Godfrey Hounsfield to produce the scanner to give the crisp detail of tumour and sensitive adjacent normal tissue, the clear body outline and a wealth of extra information on tissue densities. Positioning for treatment planning has been restricted, but now the facilities of the new generation of scanners will allow this to be improved.

The question of cost has been left to the last. There is little doubt that it costs much more in both patient suffering and money, not to mention time, to embark on a prolonged course of palliation rather than to cure a patient.

The scanner is already deeply involved in oncological practice and if the wealth of information it produces on diagnosis, staging, monitoring tumour response and for more effective treatment planning can contribute directly to the cure as opposed to the palliation of even a further small percentage of patients with cancer, then all the time and money spent will be justified.

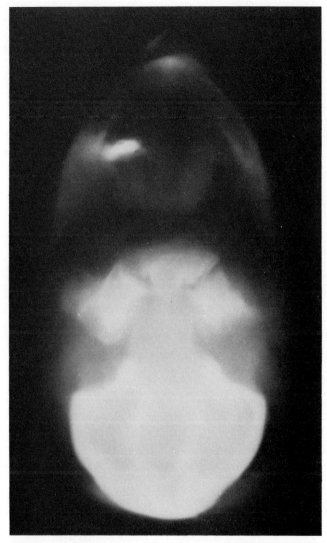

Fig. 1.4 Carcinoma of the tongue. Transverse axial tomograph through the base of the skull. A drop of barium has been placed in the ulcer on the surface of the tongue.

Acknowledgements

Grateful acknowledgement is made to the Cancer Research Campaign for the provision of an EMI 5005 General Purpose Scanner at the Royal Marsden Hospital, Surrey, and to the Department of Health and Social Security for its housing and running expenses.

8

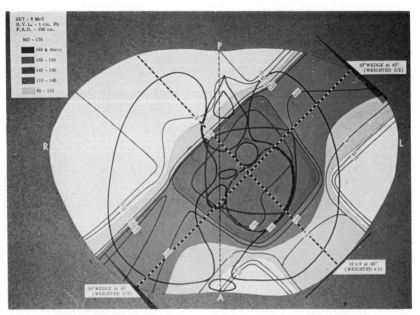

Fig. 1.5 Carcinoma of the bronchus (same patient as Fig. 1.3). Treatment plan produced from transverse axial tomographs through the level of the tumour.

References

Collins V P, Loeffler R K, Tivey H 1956 Observation on growth rates of human tumours. American Journal of Roentgenology 76: 988

Ennals D 1978 Proceedings of the Nursing Mirror International Cancer Nursing Conference. Nursing Mirror, 1–4

Hobday P A, Hodson N J, Husband J E, Parker R P, Macdonald J S 1979 Radiology 133: 477–482

Husband J E, Parker R P, Cassell K C, Hobday P A, Macdonald J S 1978 Radiation therapy planning using a CT 5005 whole body scanner. Xtract 2: 2–5

Macdonald J S, Parker R P, Husband J E, Hobday P A, Cattell A 1977 Change in patient treatment plans arising from CT scanning. Paper read at the Radiological Society of North America meeting, Chicago, December 2nd 1977

Macdonald J S 1964 Transverse axial tomography. Paper read at the Annual Meeting of the Faculty of Radiologists, June 1964

Parker R P 1979 Personal communication

Smithers D W 1960 In: A clinical prospect of the cancer problems. E & S Livingstone, Edinburgh, Ch 3, p41

Stevenson J J 1950 Horizontal body section radiography. British Journal of Radiology 23: 319–334

Watson W 1937 British Patents 508, 381

2. The present status of scanner technology

B. R. PULLAN

Introduction

Scanner technology has developed significantly since the early machine developed by Dr Godfrey Hounsfield. The developments have been largely in terms of convenience of operation and in particular in speed of computing. Increases in matrix size and improvements in display technology have produced increasingly acceptable images although some sacrifices have been made in terms of accuracy with modern fast scanners. The prototype CT scanner produced by Dr Hounsfield in 1972 is still probably the most accurate scanner made and comparable measurement accuracy is difficult to achieve with the more modern designs. The dose efficiency of this early scanner was also very high; comparable values are now being achieved with the latest technology using large display and computation matrices.

A CT scanner comprises a number of discrete elements, the technological developments in which can be considered separately. The influence of the developments upon the whole scanner performance can then be assessed. In this chapter the recent developments in technology in respect of each component will be described and possible future developments indicated. The elements which will be considered will be: the scanner configuration, the X-ray tube, the detectors, the computer and computer algorithm. The overall performance will be assessed in terms of measure of image quality and speed.

Scanner configurations

Altogether five configurations are in use at this time: the rotate translate single and fan beam scanners, the rotating detector array and source scanners, the rotating source and stationary detector, and finally the rotating source nutating detector array scanners. Only the first four of these find wide use and the single beam rotate translate scanners are rapidly becoming obsolete. The most used configurations in current machines are the rotating detector rotating X-ray tube and the rotating source stationary detector designs. These rotate only machines are illustrated in Figures 2.1 and 2.2 and have the advantages that high speed scanning can be achieved at high dose efficiency.

X-ray sources

All current rotate only machines use light rotating anode tubes and these appear to

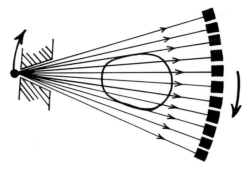

Fig. 2.1 Configuration of the rotating detector array and source scanner.

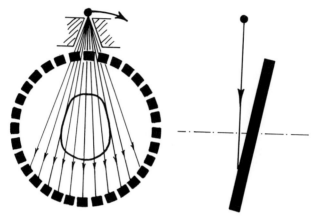

Fig. 2.2 Configuration of the nutating detector array, rotating source scanner.

be close to achievable technical limits. Calculation indicates that the limit appears to be at a useful output of 10^{14} photons/hour. This corresponds to approximately 40-50 slices per hour at currently acceptable standards of scan quality. Outputs are however such that individual scans can be taken in times of the order of one second but thermal loading sets a strict limit to the number of such scans which can be completed in any period of time.

Developments are taking place in X-ray sources in which electron beams are scanned along large semi-circular targets so producing a rapidly moving X ray source. In one such design Boyd et al (1979) propose the use of multiple target rings to allow rapid sequential visualisation of consecutive slices.

Detectors

Major advances in CT detector technology have taken place and these will continue. Current scanners appear to be using either Xenon detector arrays or modular solid state detectors employing packs of dense scintillator crystals coupled to photo diodes. One scanner design employs an array of 540 Xenon detector elements with a 1 mm spacing and the majority of rotating detector devices appear to favour the use of Xenon detectors. A particular example of a scintillator photo diode-detector module consists of an array of 8 detectors mounted on the end of a plug in module. In the scanner configuration shown in Figure 2.2, 136 of these detector modules are mounted side by side to give a very close packed and thus dose efficient ring of 1088 individual detector elements. In this particular example Caesium Iodide crystals are used with a spacing of about 1 mm. A number of possible alternative types of crystals are available with light outputs suitable for use with photo diodes and one of these, Cadmium Tungstate, may find a place in the future.

Algorithm and computing

Little development appears necessary in the basic reconstruction algorithm although more accurate and faster beam hardening corrections are required for quantitative measurement when using rotate only scanners without carefully positioned patients and bolus.

Current computing technology is capable of producing diagnostic images in times of the order of that required for data collection. Accurate corrected data takes significantly longer to compute but the introduction of array and pipeline processors will have a significant impact in this area.

Performance

This can be measured in terms of a large number of parameters but the most important are perhaps patient throughput, speed of scan, accuracy, image quality and dose efficiency.

The ultimate limit on patient throughput is set by tube output and at the limit of 40-50 slices per hour and an average of 10 slices per patient the throughput cannot exceed 4 to 5 patients per hour, if reasonable picture quality is to be achieved. Operational constraints usually limit the throughput to considerably less than the above figure.

Scan speeds as short as 1 second are obtainable on commercially available equipment and high quality scans can be achieved in routine operation with 3 second scan times. This is still not short enough to arrest heart motion and a number of interesting developments are taking place using either gating methods (Berninger et al, 1979) or fast scanners using rotating image intensifiers (Robb et al, 1979).

Image quality and dose efficiency are both related and must be considered together. There is no universally acceptable measure of image quality but two which can be related to the physical efficiency of the scanner are used widely. The first of these involves measuring the line or impulse response (using wires in a water filled phantom) at the same time as the noise (relative standard deviation of attenuation values) and maximum and integrated radiation dose are measured. The width of the impulse response at half height w, the maximum radiation dose D, and the relative standard deviation σ are related by the following expression:

$$D = \frac{K_1}{\sigma^2 \times w^3}$$

the constant, K_1, depends upon the particular object being scanned and for good current technology has a value of about 1.7 for a 20 cm diameter water bath when

12

w is measured in millimetres, D in rads and σ is expressed as a percentage of the attenuation value for water. This is quite close to the ultimate limit set by the physics and statistics of the method and typical values of D, w and σ for a 20 cm diameter water phantom would be 2 rads, 1.5 mm and 0.5 per cent respectively.

The second method of measuring image quality makes use of contrast perception diagrams. In this method a phantom is used in which pins of different diameter and different contrast relative to the background is scanned and the pin which can just be detected by a set of observers determined. A graph is then plotted of the logarithm of the contrast, C per cent, which can just be detected for a given pin diameter against the logarithm of pin diameter, d. Over a reasonable range of pin sizes and contrasts, values fall on a straight line the position of which depends upon dose, D. Two such straight lines are shown plotted in Figure 2.3. The lines can be described by a simple equation as follows:

$$dC \sqrt{D} = K_2$$

For pins placed in a 20 cm diameter water bath the value of K_2 is in the range 3.0 − 4.0 with good current technology and again this is close to the physically achievable limits.

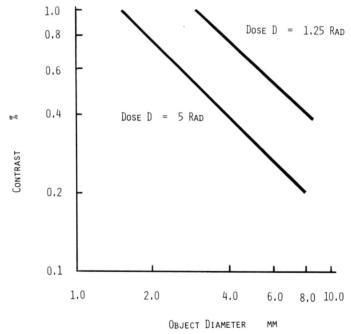

Fig. 2.3 Contrast perception diagram, shown for doses of 1.25 and 5 rads.

Developments

A recent development has been the scout view or scannogram in which the detectors of a scanner are used to gather data to produce a plain radiograph of the patient. In a good scanner, this is achieved at a dose efficiency close to the theoretical limit and when used with contrast agents and image subtraction or other forms of image processing scannogram may find much wider application than the simple patient positioning for which they are primarily intended.

Rapid developments are also taking place in emission CT using radioactive isotopes. Excellent representations of the distribution of metabolism and function have been demonstrated using positron emission tomography. Whilst the requirement of a local cyclotron to make full use of these scanners will probably limit their use to research activity in most countries of the world, the latest results with single photon emission tomography are excellent. The wider availability of I ^{123} and other reasonably long-lived accelerator produced isotopes combined with these developments could lead to exciting advances in functional imaging.

Some of the more promising N.M.R. imaging methods also employ CT reconstruction techniques and the recent developments in this field combined with its probably very low levels of hazard promise a very important future.

References

Berninger W H, Redinton R W, Doherty P, Lipton M H, Carlsson E 1979 Gated cardiac scanning: canine studies. Journal of Computer Assisted Tomography 3(2): 155–163

Boyd D P, Gould R G, Quinn J R, Sparks R, Stanley J H, Herrmannsfeldt W B 1979 IEEE Transactions on Nuclear Science NS-26 (No. 2 April 1979): 2724–2727

Robb R A, Ritman E L, Gilbert B K, Kinsey J H, Harris L D, Wood E H 1979 The D.S.R.: a high speed three dimensional X-ray computed tomography system for dynamic spatial reconstruction of the heart and circulation. IEEE Transactions on Nuclear Science NS-26 (No. 2 April 1979): 2713–2717

3. The role of CT in primary diagnosis—an overview

I. KELSEY FRY

The role of CT in the staging and management of malignant disease is obvious. CT of the body is, however, seriously undervalued if it is thought of essentially as an aid to the management of known malignant disease. Its uses can be considered under four headings:

1. Primary diagnosis
2. Assessment and follow up of known benign disease
3. Determination of stage and extent of known malignancy
4. Radiotherapy treatment planning.

To me as a general clinical radiologist it is the diagnostic scans which seem the most immediately rewarding in terms of patient care. Improved staging and improved radiotherapy treatment planning can be expected to improve the outcome of disease but some years must elapse before such benefits can be established. Benefits obtained from more accurate, more comprehensive, less hazardous and more comfortable primary diagnosis are more easily recognised in the short term.

How useful is CT in primary diagnosis? In particular, how useful is it in the primary diagnosis of malignant disease? In order to obtain information which might help to answer these questions one thousand consecutive body scans carried out at St Bartholomew's Hospital have been reviewed. St Bartholomew's is an 850 bedded general teaching hospital with a major oncology unit and an active radiotherapy department. A separate scanner is available for brain scans. All the scans were done using an EMI 5005 scanner with a scan time of 18-20 seconds.

The patients were divided into three groups with indications for CT as follows:
1. Primary diagnosis
2. Assessment and follow up of benign lesions
3. Diagnosis and management of known malignant disease (Table 3.1). The table shows that over 40 per cent of scans were done in patients who were not known to have malignant disease at the time of the scan.

Table 3.1 CT problems in 1000 patients

Primary diagnosis	326
Assessment or follow up of benign lesions	89
Diagnosis and management of malignancy	585

The group of patients known to have malignant disease included all the patients with a history of malignancy, however far in the past. Some of these presented with diagnostic problems which were not necessarily related to their previous disease. If such patients are added to those in whom the scans were done for primary diagnosis, approximately 40 per cent of all scans were carried out for diagnostic purposes, even in a hospital with major oncology and radiotherapy departments.

Of the 326 patients scanned for primary diagnosis, 83 presented with no suspicion of malignant disease (Fig. 3.1). The largest number (28) in this group

Fig. 3.1

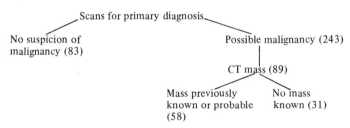

was patients with suspected intra-abdominal sepsis, one of the best indications for CT. Other indications included trauma, lesions of the renal tract including the evaluation of transplant kidneys, lesions of the spine and vascular abnormalities. The remaining 243 patients presented with symptoms and signs which might have proved to be due to malignant disease although in many instances this was unlikely. In such patients CT has two main functions. Firstly, it may confirm the presence of or show the site of and sometimes the nature of a mass suspected either by clinical examination or by another imaging technique. Secondly, it may demonstrate a mass when physical examination and other investigations have been normal or unsuccessful, or when CT is the investigation of first choice as in possible tumours of the adrenal and in some suspected abdominal masses.

Masses were shown in 89 patients, in 58 of whom CT confirmed a mass previously shown or strongly suspected on other evidence. The distribution of lesions at different sites is shown in Table 3.2. As expected, the largest groups were masses in the pancreas and mediastinum. The series included a number of scans in suspected pelvic masses. We rarely scan now for primary diagnosis in pelvic disease because in our experience CT makes little or no contribution to the diagnosis, presumably because the pelvis is more easily accessible to physical examination than the rest of the abdomen.

Table 3.2 58 patients in whom CT confirmed known or suspected mass

Pancreas	16	Kidney	3
Mediastinum	11	Aneurysm, liver, gall bladder	2 each
Pelvis	9		
Para-aortic nodes	6	Spleen, retroperitoneal sarcoma	1 each
Abdominal abscess	5		

Follow up was available in 54 patients of whom 15 proved to have malignant disease, 5 in the pancreas, 4 in lymph nodes, 2 in the mediastinum and 1 each in the liver, pelvis and retroperitoneal tissues.

CT is not tissue specific and a firm diagnosis of malignancy can rarely be made from the CT scan alone unless there are metastases or there is local spread of the disease. CT can however on occasions show that a lesion is extremely unlikely to be malignant by showing that it is cystic or contains fat or that it is an abscess. Sometimes a mass proves to be an enlarged 'normal' structure such as gall bladder, spleen or an aortic aneurysm. Thus, CT indicated the benign nature of the abnormality in 20 of the 39 patients with benign lesions, 5 in the mediastinum, 2 each in the kidney, pancreas, pelvis and gall bladder, one in the liver, 2 aneurysms of the aorta and 4 abscesses in the abdomen.

CT is shown at its most effective in the mediastinum where the demonstration that a mass seen on chest X-ray is cystic or contains fat avoids the need for further investigation. Likewise the demonstration that a wide mediastinal shadow is due simply to an excess of fat or can be accounted for by vessels is frequently reassuring. CT is also very effective in those patients with renal masses in whom ultrasound findings are equivocal. Cysts are readily distinguished from tumours.

The most interesting patients from the point of view of primary diagnosis of malignancy are the 31 in whom CT detected a mass when other investigations had not shown a mass or in whom CT was obviously the investigation of first choice. The distribution of lesions in this group is shown in Table 3.3. As expected almost all of the lesions were in the retroperitoneum, the great majority being in the pancreas, adrenals or lymph nodes.

Follow up was available in 29 patients. 17 proved to have malignant disease, 8 in lymph nodes, 4 in the pancreas, 2 in the adrenals and one each in the lung the kidney and the stomach. There were no false positives.

Table 3.3 31 patients with masses on CT previously undiagnosed

Abdominal nodes	10
Adrenals	9
Pancreas	6
Mediastinum	2
Other retroperitoneal mass	1
Kidney, lung, stomach	1 each

The patients who were investigated because of undiagnosed illness which might have been due to malignant disease included a group of 6 patients with para-aortic lymphadenopathy in whom there were no other enlarged nodes. Three of these proved to be due to Hodgkin's disease, two had metastases from unsuspected bronchial carcinoma and one had tuberculosis. Three had no sign localising disease to the abdomen. This group is important because there is a tendency to discourage the use of CT in the absence of some more localising signs. CT can, however, be of value in patients who are ill with PUO, raised ESR, weight loss etc. even when there are no symptoms or signs localising the disease to the abdomen.

Four of the pancreatic lesions were in the tail of the gland which is frequently difficult to evaluate by ultrasound. Indeed, lesions in the left upper quadrant are particularly difficult to demonstrate by standard techniques but are well suited to CT which can show all the structures in the cross section including the spleen, the tail of the pancreas, splenic hilar nodes, the kidney, the adrenal as well as masses spreading from the stomach.

CT is highly accurate at demonstrating masses in the adrenals provided they are more than 1.5–2 cm in diameter. It is the investigation of first choice in patients with Cushing's syndrome, suggested phaeochromocytoma or virilising tumour. In the study, 2 of the tumours in patients with Cushing's syndrome proved to be malignant. Conn's tumours are often too small to visualise using 18–20 second scanners but even so, CT may still be the investigation of first choice in patients with Conn's syndrome in order to detect the occasional large tumour and thus avoid more elaborate investigations. In phaeochromocytoma, scans are continued down to the aortic bifurcation and in one patient, in this study of para-aortic phaeochromocytoma, were shown at the level of L_3.

One of the mediastinal lesions was a thymoma in a patient with myasthenia gravis which in retrospect could just be seen high in the mediastinum in the lateral chest film almost completely hidden by overlying soft tissue. The other mediastinal lesion was an ACTH secreting thymic tumour lying in front of the main pulmonary artery in a patient with Cushing's syndrome associated with ectopic ACTH secretions. The lesion had not been detected in spite of repeated chest film and tomograms and could not be seen even in retrospect probably because it lay low in the anterior mediastinum close to the heart shadow.

The one renal lesion in this group was a carcinoma in a patient with pyrexia of unknown origin, raised ESR and right upper quadrant pain. CT occasionally shows quite large renal masses not demonstrated on urography because they rise from the anterior or posterior surface of the kidney and produce little calyceal distortion or deformity of outline on the straight A-P view of the abdomen.

The lung lesion was a 1.5 cm primary carcinoma in a patient with a positive sputum but normal chest film and tomography and a negative bronchoscopy. The lesion in the stomach was a carcinoma in a hiatus hernia. It had not been detected on a barium meal six months earlier: a CT scan was done when the patient continued to lose weight.

It is interesting to observe that of the 246 patients scanned for primary diagnosis in whom the presentation raised the possibility of malignant disease, a diagnosis of malignancy was established in 32 and that in more than half of these no mass had been demonstrated before CT.

As already stated, CT alone cannot usually determine the precise nature of a mass of soft tissue density. It is however an excellent method for guiding percutaneous biopsy. Its use for this purpose overlaps that of ultrasound. The choice will depend on personal experience and availability of the appropriate equipment. CT is more precise and is particularly useful for small lesions especially those in the retroperitoneum.

So far I have discussed those patients in whom CT has shown a mass. In some ways even more effective is its ability to exclude the presence of a mass which is suspected on physical examination or by some other imaging technique. Its effectiveness in this context illustrates two of the three great advantages of CT as an imaging technique (Table 3.4). Firstly, CT is not organ specific. As already discussed in relation to the left upper quadrant, CT demonstrates all the structures in the

Table 3.4 Special features of CT of the body

1. Not organ specific

2. Credibility high

3. Minimal operator dependence

cross section. The referring clinician does not have to choose an appropriate imaging technique to outline each organ in turn. In the case of a suspected mass one can be sure that, whatever its suspected source, it would be included in the scan. Secondly, and perhaps more important, the credibility of CT is high. The images are relatively easily understood by an untrained observer so that the clinician finds the report relatively easy to accept as a basis for decisions on management. Because of the high credibility a negative CT scan frequently has more value than is usual with other imaging techniques. It is, for instance, particularly valuable for excluding a mass in the abdomen when clinical examination is equivocal.

The third special feature of the CT is the fact that unlike ultrasound it is dependent on the skill of the operator to a minimum degree.

Within the abdomen ultrasound and CT may appear to compete. There is no question of competition. The techniques are complementary. Whenever possible ultrasound should be used first because it is quicker, cheaper, carries no radiation hazard and is more pleasant for the patient. The two machines should be situated close together. In situations where both techniques are applicable such as the liver, pancreas and kidney ultrasound/CT should be regarded as one diagnostic package. CT will be indicated only when ultrasound is unsuccessful or equivocal or if the clinician requires confirmation of the ultrasound findings.

The major indications for a CT in primary diagnosis are summarised in Table 3.5.

Table 3.5 Major indications for CT in primary diagnosis

Mediastinum

   site of mass
   nature of mass
   occult disease

Adrenals

Pancreas (US/CT)

Abdominal sepsis (US/CT)

Abdominal masses especially when equivocal (US/CT)

Suspected retroperitoneal lesions

This discussion has concentrated on those patients in whom CT might have made contribution to the diagnosis of malignant disease. The study of another diagnostic situation such as trauma, abdominal sepsis, abnormalities of the lungs, spine and other tissues or vascular abnormalities has only been briefly touched upon. As machines become more widely available and the potential of the method is appreciated by clinicians so its use for diagnostic purposes will increase. Difficulties will arise as to the proper distribution of scanning time between scans for diagnosis and those for the management of malignant disease. The resolution of such difficulties will require nice judgement. Our task as radiologists is to provide our clinical colleagues with as much information as possible so that the technique can be used to best advantage.

4. Pancreatic cancer—computed tomography versus ultrasound and conventional techniques

CLAUS D. CLAUSSEN, OTTO H. WEGNER and MARTIN PFISTER

Introduction

In recent years the incidence of pancreatic carcinoma has risen in the industrial countries; in Japan the mortality rate of pancreatic carcinoma has risen approximately six times from 1951 to 1972 (Ariyama & Shirakabe, 1979). The disease now accounts for 3 per cent of all cancers and 5 per cent of cancer deaths in the United States (Hermann & Cooperman, 1979). Pancreatic carcinoma is now the fourth most commonest cause of death from cancer in men (1. lung 2. colorectal 3. prostate) and the fifth in women (1. breast 2. colorectal 3. lung 4. ovary/uterus).

Numerous reports of invasive and non-invasive methods for diagnosing pancreatic carcinoma have been published and have been largely confined to diagnostic accuracy of the different techniques available. However, treatment has not resulted in a better prognosis – the overall five-year survival rate is less than 1 per cent (Aoki & Ogawa, 1978). One of the reasons for this is that there are neither specific initial symptoms in patients with pancreatic carcinoma nor any simple immuno-serological examinations for clinical screening to diagnose the disease at an early localised stage. Few reports deal with the relationship of the size and location of the pancreatic carcinoma to the diagnostic accuracy or to resectability.

Improved therapeutic results in pancreatic carcinoma will not occur if only the large and unresectable tumours are diagnosed. Approximately 85 to 90 per cent of pancreatic cancers have extended beyond the pancreas or metastases are present at the time of operative exploration (Cubilla et al, 1978).

The pancreas is acknowledged to be a difficult organ to evaluate both by clinical and routine radiological methods. Even with the development of invasive and the new non-invasive methods. such as ultrasound and computed tomography (CT), the detection of small carcinomas of the pancreas is very difficult. Both CT and ultrasound provide the facility to image the pancreatic parenchyma directly. With the introduction of CT there was great hope that this technique would open the way to more precise and earlier diagnosis of pancreatic cancer.

The purpose of this chapter is to give a critical appraisal of the use of CT in the investigation of pancreatic cancer and, as far as possible to compare this technique with other methods of investigation, especially ultrasound. The limitations of the methods and the diagnostic criteria used in evaluating the pancreas will be discussed.

Technique of examination and anatomic considerations

The pancreas can usually be well demonstrated by CT. In the literature the success rate in identifying the gland reaches between 92 and 98 per cent. With the development of new fast high resolution scanners this is likely to rise to almost 100 per cent (Sheedy et al, 1977; Hessel et al, 1979). With ultrasound the pancreas is identified less frequently, detection rates have ranged from 65 to 90 per cent (Filly & Stuart, 1979; de Graff & Taylor, 1978).

Air in the gastrointestinal tract is one of the most important limiting factors with ultrasound, preventing complete or partial visualisation of the pancreas in approximately 10 to 15 per cent of patients. Visualisation of the tail is particularly difficult; however, using CT good visualisation of the tail is usually achieved. Obesity is a further major disadvantage with ultrasound whereas thin patients are difficult to evaluate with CT.

One of the main advantages of CT is that it is not organ specific, a good survey of the topographical and anatomic relations of all the organs within the cross-section is provided. Furthermore, standardisation of the examination with CT is easier than with ultrasound. No special bowel preparation programme is required. Generally the patient is given a dilute water soluble contrast medium orally (gastrografin 2 to 5 per cent) 30 to 45 minutes before the examination. Using an 18 second scanner a smooth muscle relaxant, such as glucagon or buscopan, is also given (Sheedy et al, 1977; Lee et al, 1979; Moss et al, 1978).

Opacification of the pancreatic parenchyma is now being undertaken in those centres where high resolution sub-5 second scanners are available (Marchal et al, 1979). Enhancement of the normal parenchyma may permit small intrapancreatic tumours to be identified as areas of lower attenuation (Marshall et al, 1979). During the scan respiration must be suspended to reduce motion artefacts.

Examination of the normal pancreas has demonstrated that the pancreas varies considerably in its size, shape and location in the upper retroperitoneal abdomen. The organ can be more easily identified in patients with ample retroperitoneal fat because the fat surrounds the outlines of the gland. In very thin patients the margins can be difficult to define.

Using an 18 second scanner and 13 mm thick slices, the pancreas usually appears smooth and homogeneous in density but in 20 to 30 per cent of patients the organ is lobulated (Ferrucci et al, 1979). Occasionally, the lower part of the pancreatic head, the uncinate process, stands in a 'hook-like fashion' lateral and posterior to the mesenteric vein. The caudal portion may lie in the section of the left renal vein (Stephens, 1979).

Haaga et al (1977) compared the thickness of the different parts of the pancreas with the second lumbar vertebral body. The head of the pancreas should not be greater in size than the full transverse diameter. The body and tail should not be greater than two-thirds of this vertebral body. Kreel et al (1977) also measured the dimensions of the normal pancreas. Their measurements, based on scans taken using an 18 second scanner, were different from those of Haaga et al (1979). (Maximum anterior-posterior dimensions in the supine position 3 cm head, 2.5 cm neck and body and 2 cm tail).

The size of the pancreas is variable and decreases with age. Alterations in contour of the normal pancreas are usually gradual rather than abrupt. When there is little retroperitoneal fat the organs may form a composite image thus simulating a mass. In this situation, if a mass in the pancreatic head is suspected we usually repeat the examination in the right lateral decubitus position.

Criteria used in the diagnosis of pancreatic pathology

Using CT, it is generally possible to detect a pancreatic mass which alters the contour of the gland. Recognition of abrupt transition of the contour is more important than absolute measurements of size (Stephens, 1979). With the new generation of fast scanners it is nearly always possible to identify partial or diffuse enlargement. In our opinion, the diagnostic dilemma is that there are no specific absorption values for neoplastic or inflammatory tissue; inflammatory and malignant tissue may have the same density measurements as normal pancreatic parenchyma. Lower absorption patterns can be a sign of oedema which is often seen in combination with inflammatory disease, or with necrosis of a tumour (Sheedy et al, 1977).

Malignant tumours of the pancreas are most commonly adenocarcinomas; cystadenocarcinomas are relatively rare. Nearly two-thirds of pancreatic cancers are localised in the head of the gland; these have a slightly better prognosis than those localised in the body and tail because obstructive jaundice tends to be a relatively early presenting feature (Hermann and Cooperman, 1979).

Solid lesions have no specific typical morphology and are only recognised because they produce enlargement. There is usually an abrupt change in pancreatic contour at the junction of the mass with normal tissue and lesions are commonly only recognised if greater than 3 cm in diameter. Intrapancreatic tumours, which do not change the size and shape of the gland, are not detectable.

In contrast to malignant lesions of the liver, the tissue density of pancreatic carcinomas is usually indistinguishable from that of normal pancreatic parenchyma, except when a hypodense area due to necrosis is seen (Sheedy et al, 1977). Small tumours can only be identified if they arise from the surface of the gland or are located in the uncinate process. Tumours here, produce rounded ovoid borders of the anterior and posterior surfaces of the uncinate process and a loss of the 'hook-shaped' extension behind the superior mesenteric vein (Lee et al, 1979).

With ultrasound, carcinomas appear as mass lesions with a decreased number of irregularly distributed internal echoes. This is accepted as one of the most important criteria for diagnosis of pancreatic malignancy (Weinstein et al, 1979). However, specific patterns indicating a benign or malignant lesion have not yet been described and chronic pancreatitis remains a 'shadow' of pancreatic cancer (Sample, 1979). In practice, in both our experience and that of others (Ferrucci et al, 1979) a non-calcified mass due to chronic pancreatitis cannot be distinguished from a pancreatic neoplasm either with ultrasound or with CT.

Extension of a pancreatic carcinoma into surrounding tissues produces obliteration of retropancreatic fat around the superior mesenteric artery and is an important diagnostic sign of pancreatic carcinoma (Haaga et al, 1977; Friedmann, 1979; Modder et al, 1979; Lackner et al, 1979).

Sometimes a pancreatic carcinoma is associated with inflammation and then the margins of the gland are not clearly defined. It is usually possible to make a definitive diagnosis of carcinoma of the pancreas with CT if secondary signs of malignancy are present. These include dilatation of the common bile ducts and/or intrahepatic bile ducts or the pancreatic duct. These features may be the only evidence of a carcinoma of the head. Fishman et al (1979) report a 2 per cent incidence of dilatation of the pancreatic duct in a study of CT in patients with suspected pancreatic disease. The dilated duct is seen as a linear water density structure throughout the length of the gland. Dilatation of the pancreatic duct and/or the common bile duct is also seen in pancreatitis (Fishman et al, 1979). Unequivocal signs of a malignant pancreatic mass are metastases in the liver and enlargement of the peripancreatic and retroperitoneal lymph nodes.

In accordance with several other reports nearly half the patients in which a dilated duct was demonstrated were suffering from chronic pancreatitis and the other half from carcinoma. This finding of a dilated duct thus confirms the presence of pancreatic disease but is not specific for a neoplasm. Calcification in the pancreas may be seen in carcinomas as well as pancreatitis. Ferrucci et al (1979) describe two patients with pancreatic carcinoma in which calcification was demonstrated within the tumour. In addition, they found a 4 per cent incidence of pancreatic cancer occurring in association with chronic calcareous pancreatitis.

Discussion

There is no doubt that the success rate of detecting cancers with CT using the new fast scanners is nearly 100 per cent, but there are many more unsuccessful examinations using ultrasound. A review of the current literature regarding the diagnostic accuracy of CT in the diagnosis of pancreatic cancer gives the surprising result that there are only a few cases of carcinoma which are not detected with CT (Sheedy et al, 1977; Husband et al, 1977; Haaga et al, 1977; Levitt et al, 1978; Lawson et al, 1979; Lackner et al, 1979). All these reports give a description of the typical findings in pancreatic carcinoma but the number of cases where the results have been compared with other methods of investigation are low. The reports do not give specific information about the size of the detected carcinomas. In our experience most pancreatic carcinomas diagnosed by CT are large and could well be identified by other diagnostic methods. The largest series (Haaga et al, 1977; Sheedy et al, 1977; Hessel et al, 1979; Stanley et al, 1977) report an overall accuracy of 83, 88, 90 and 94 per cent respectively. In addition, the sensitivity of detecting pancreatic carcinoma is high 83, 88 and 94 per cent (Lackner et al, 1979; Sheedy et al, 1977) while the sensitivity of CT in detecting pancreatitis is much lower 56, 69 and 81 per cent (Ferrucci et al, 1979). It is interesting to note that most authors who have reported the results of the accuracy of ultrasound have a similar sensitivity rate as with CT and occasionally a higher accuracy (Fineberg et al; Barkin et al, 1977). However, Ferrucci et al (1979) and Levitt et al (1978) in a prospective study report a significantly lower sensitivity and accuracy using ultrasound compared with CT. On the other hand, Weill et al (1977) report 95 per cent accuracy using ultrasound in the detection of pancreatic disease, but in this series there was no comparison made with CT.

In our opinion there is no doubt that in cases undergoing both CT and ultrasound, ultrasound gives considerably less information than CT. The advantages of CT are (a) better visualisation of the pancreas and (b) physicians, with little CT experience, are able to interpret the CT images.

Thus, CT would appear to be the most effective method for detecting pancreatic carcinoma. However, without the secondary signs of malignancy (liver metastases, retroperitoneal and peripancreatic lymph node enlargement and dilatation of the bile and pancreatic ducts) there are no absolute CT criteria for distinguishing an inflammatory mass from a neoplasm (Friedmann, 1979). If there is focal enlargement of the gland, then it is only possible to give a probability diagnosis.

Stephens (1979) discusses some of the problems of CT in the diagnosis of pancreatic carcinoma. The exact incidence of false negative examinations is not yet known since relatively few patients with normal CT scans have undergone surgical exploration and follow up periods are still short. A further source of error is that extrinsic pancreatic masses may be misinterpreted as arising in the pancreas itself. This may be a particular problem if there is invasion of the extrinsic mass into the pancreas. As previously mentioned, one of the major difficulties is the distinction of a carcinoma from chronic pancreatitis; in the series reported by Ferrucci et al (1979) scans were reported as an indeterminate (cancer/inflammation) in 24 per cent.

The relative roles of endoscopic retrograde pancreatography (ERCP), percutaneous angiography and angiography in the diagnosis of pancreatic carcinoma are beyond the scope of this text. However, a combination of these techniques, although invasive, can provide high diagnostic accuracy (Ariyama & Shirakabe, 1979).

No imaging technique can replace histological diagnosis. Both ultrasound and CT are increasingly being used for percutaneous fine needle aspiration (Fuchs et al, 1980).

Conclusion

Although there are advantages and limitations to every diagnostic imaging modality, we recommend the following scheme as a reference in the diagnostic procedure of patients with suspected pancreatic disease. These views correspond to those of Stanley & Sagel (1979).

1. If there is a low clinical index of suspicion of pancreatic disease ultrasound should be the method of choice because of the low cost and absence of radiation.

2. If there is a high index of suspicion of pancreatic disease, especially carcinoma, CT is the method of choice if the technique is available. In addition, the precise site and size of the lesion can be assessed for radiotherapy planning purposes and for monitoring therapeutic response (Kreel, 1979).

3. If a mass is found either by CT or ultrasound percutaneous fine needle aspiration biopsy should be undertaken.

4. If the results of CT and ultrasound are equivocal then more invasive methods should be used, e.g. endoscopic retrograde pancreatico-cholangiography, percutaneous transhepatic cholangiography (PTC) or angiography.

References

Aoki K, Ogawa H 1978 Cancer of the pancreas. International mortality trends. World Health Statistical Report 31 (2): 2–27

Ariyama J, Shirakabe H 1979 The diagnosis of small resectable pancreatic carcinoma. 4th European Congress of Radiology, Hamburg

Barkin J, Vining D, Miale A Jr, Gottlibe S, Redlhammer D E, Kalser M H 1977 Computerised tomography, diagnostic ultrasound and radionuclide scanning: comparison of efficacy in diagnosis of pancreatic carcinoma. Journal of the American Medical Association 238: 2040

Boijsen E 1979 Angiographic procedures in pancreatic disease. 4th European Congress of Radiology, Hamburg

Claussen C, Fischer E, Menges V, Lange D, Schenck P 1976 The value of pancreas nuclear isotope scanning in the clinical diagnostic procedure. In: Hofer (ed) Radioaktive Isotope in Klinik und Forschung 12. Egerman, Wien, p 115–126

Cubilla A L, Fortner J, Fitzgerald P J 1978 Lymph node involvement in carcinoma of the head of the pancreas area. Cancer 41: 880–887

De Graff C S, Taylor K J W, Simmonds B D, Puosenfield A T 1978 Gray scale echography of the pancreas: re-evaluation of normal size. Radiology 129: 157–161

Ferrucci J T Jr, Wittenberg J, Black E B, Kirkpatrick R H, Hall D A 1979 Computed body tomography in chronic pancreatitis. Radiology 130: 175–182

Filly R A, Stuart S L 1979 The normal pancreas: acoustic characteristics and frequency of imaging. Journal of Clinical Ultrasound 7: 121–124

Fishman A, Isikoff M B, Barkin J S, Friedland J T 1979 Significance of a dilated pancreatic duct on CT examination. American Journal of Roentgenology 133: 225–227

Friedmann G 1979 Signifikanz radiologischer Methoden der Diagnostik der Pankreaserkrankungen. Ergebnisse der Computertomographie. 4th European Congress of Radiology, Hamburg

Fuchs W, Vock P, Haertell M 1980 CT guided aspiration biopsies. Proceedings of the European Seminar on Computed Tomography in Oncology, London

Haaga J R, Alfidi R J, Havrilla T R, Tubbs R, Gonzalez L, Meaney T F, Corsi M A 1977 Definitive role of CT scanning of the pancreas. Radiology 124: 723

Haaga J R, Reich N E, Havrilla T R, Alfidi R J, Meaney T F 1977 CT guided biopsy. Cleveland Clinics Q 44: 1

Hermann R E, Cooperman A M 1979 Current concepts in cancer. Cancer of the pancreas. New England Journal of Medicine 301(9): 482–485

Hessel S J, Seigelmann S S, Adams D F, Sanders R C, McNeil B J, Alderson P N, Finberg H J, Abrams H L 1979 Prospective analysis of computed tomography and ultrasound in evaluating the pancreas. 65th Scientific Assembly of the Radiological Society of North America, Atlanta

Husband J E, Meire H B, Kreel L 1977 Comparison of ultrasound and computer-assisted tomography in pancreatic diagnosis. British Journal of Radiology 50: 855–862

Kreel L 1979 Medical imaging. H M & M Publishers, Aylesbury

Kreel L, Haertel M, Katz D 1977 Computed tomography of the normal pancreas. Journal of Computer Assisted Tomography 1: 290–299

Lackner K H, Frommhold H, Granthoff H, Modder U, Heuser L, Braun G, Buurman R, Schere K 1979 Wertigkeit der Computertomographie und Sonographie innerhalb der Pankreasdiagnostik. 4th European Congress of Radiology, Hamburg

Lawson T L, Foley W D, Stewart E T 1979 Comparative efficacy of ultrasound, computed tomography and endoscopic retrograde cholangio-pancreatography in the diagnosis of pancreatic disease. 65th Scientific Assembly of the Radiological Society of North America, Atlanta

Lee J K, Stanely R J, Melson G L, Sagel S S 1979 Pancreatic imaging by ultrasound and computed tomography. Radiological Clinics of North America 17(1): 105–117

Levitt R G, Geiss G, Sagel S S, Stanley R J, Evens R G, Koehler R E, Jost R G 1978 Complementary use of ultrasound and computed tomography in studies of the pancreas and kidney. Radiology 126: 149–152

Marchal G, Baert A L, Wilms G 1979 Intravenous pancreaticography in computed tomography. Journal of Computer Assisted Tomography 3(6): 727–732

Modder U, Friedmann G, Bucheler E, Baert E, Lackner C, Brecht G, Buurmann R, Rupp N, Heller H J 1979 Wert und Ergebnisse der Computertomographie bei Pankreaserkrankungen. Fortschritte Rontgenstrahlen 130(1): 57–61

Moss A A, Kressel H Y, Korobkin M, Goldberg H I, Rohlfing B M, Brasch R C 1978 The effect of gastrografin and glucagon on CT scanning of the pancreas: a blind clinical trial. Radiology 126: 711–714

Ponette E, Pringot J, Baert A L, Marchal G, Dardene A N, Goenen Y 1976 Computerised tomography and ultrasonography in pancreatitis. Acta Gastroenterologie Belgium 39: 402

Sample W F 1979 Pancreatic mass ultrasound. In: Moss A A, Goldberg H J (eds) Computed tomography ultrasound and X-ray: an integrated approach. Masson, New York, 457–468

Sheedy P F, Stephens D H, Hattery R R, MacCarty R 1977 Computed tomography in the evaluation of patients with suspected carcinoma of the pancreas. Radiology 124: 731–737

Stanley R J, Sagel S S 1979 Computed tomography of the pancreas. Syllabus categorical course in computed tomography. 65th Scientific Assembly and Annual Meeting, Radiological Society of North America, Atlanta

Stanley R J, Sagel S S, Levitt R G 1977 Computed tomography evaluation of the pancreas. Radiology 124: 715–722

Stephens D H 1979 Pancreatic mass computed tomography. In: Moss A A, Goldberg H J (eds) Computed tomography, ultrasound and X-ray: an integrated approach. Masson, New York, 469–479

Weill F, Schraub A, Eisenscher A, Bourgoin A 1977 Ultrasonography of the normal pancreas. Radiology 123: 417–423

Weinstein D P, Wolfmann N T, Weinstein B J 1979 Ultrasonic characteristics of pancreatic tumours. Gastro Radiology 4: 245–251

5. CT-guided aspiration techniques

W. A. FUCHS, P. VOCK and M. HAERTEL

Guidance on needle procedures is achieved by various techniques and selecting the most suitable mainly depends on the localisation of the pathological process. Sampling of superficial lesions in the breast, lymph nodes, and prostate is usually done by direct vision. A high rate of positive tissue sampling by fluoroscopically guided aspiration of pulmonary neoplasm has been proven in a large series of cases. Fluoroscopy and CT are both valuable tools in directing needles for the biopsy of mediastinal pathology. Ultrasound and CT are the two methods of choice for needle guidance in the abdominal area.

The transverse plane of computed tomography accurately displays both the normal anatomy and the specific topographic localisation of pathological lesions and therefore enables the accurate percutaneous placement of biopsy needles.

Puncture techniques

A diagnostic computed tomogram is essential to demonstrate and localise the pathological lesion prior to any CT guided biopsy. The diagnostic CT cut that best demonstrates the pathological area must be reset with the patient holding his breath in deep inspiration. The tentative entry point of the biopsy needle is then chosen within that slice. The needle path should ideally correspond to the shortest distance from the body surface to the mass lesion. Bony elements, blood vessels and nerves should, however, be avoided. Accurate needle positioning is easily determined and achieved in the horizontal X-axis and vertical Y-axis, since its direction and depth can be accurately calculated on the anatomic slice on the CT monitor. The sagittal Z-axis accuracy is defined by the 8 - 10 mm anatomic slice thickness (Fig. 5.1). Diversion of the needle from the ideal sagittal plane occurs when the direction of the needle path is angulated, that is, when the biopsy needle passes obliquely through the plane of the CT scan. The point at which the needle passes out of the plane of the CT control scan may be interpreted as the needle tip, whereas in fact the tip is actually situated somewhere outside that plane. Such problems of needle positioning mainly occur in biopsy of deeply-seated lesions when using fine flexible, easily deflexible needles. A small amount of contrast material may be injected during the biopsy procedure to identify the actual site of the biopsy (Stephenson et al, 1979). Depending on the topographic anatomical localisation of the lesion, the patient may be turned from the supine to a lateral decubital or prone position. A control CT scan is then taken with skin markers, a lead pellet, and a needle or a marking frame, to reveal the exact site of

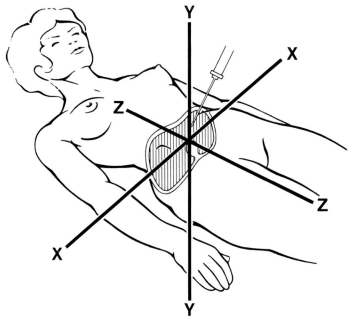

Fig. 5.1 Placement of biopsy needle with relationship to the horizontal (X), vertical (Y) and sagittal plane (Z) (according to Haaga, 1979).

the point of entry (Fig. 5.2). If the entry point is satisfactory, the chosen site is draped in a sterile fashion and a local anaesthetic administered. The percutaneous insertion and positioning of the needle may be performed according to various techniques.

A free-handed needle technique is applied to puncture large and superficially located mass lesions. The position of skin markers relative to the mass lesion, visualised on the monitor, determines both the angle of direction as well as the depth of puncture. The needle is then inserted free-handed, according to the 'position feeling' of the investigator, up to the previously marked distance. The exact position of the needle tip is then verified by a control scan after moving the patient into the exact position within the gantry. If the localisation of the needle tip is not satisfactory, further positioning is necessary to place the needle tip within the area to be investigated.

With the *coaxial double needle puncture technique,* (Fig. 5.3) a large bore 18 gauge needle with an outer diameter of 1.2 mm is introduced into the trunk wall and a repeat scan is obtained. If the needle is properly directed towards the lesion, a 22 gauge (0.9 mm) needle may then be advanced through the 18 gauge needle to the predetermined depth. Now the patient is moved back into the scanning gantry and a repeat scan is obtained to verify the position of the needle tip. This technique is advantageous inasmuch as the patient feels the pain of the skin perforation only once. In addition, a fine calibre needle may be inserted without resistance and without changing direction, thereby allowing multiple punctures without difficulty.

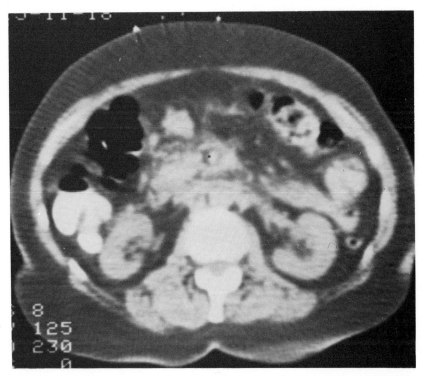

Fig. 5.2 Control scan with lead pellets to mark the entry point for biopsy of carcinoma of the head of the pancreas.

For the purpose of multiple punctures the so-called *tandem* or parallel needle technique may be applied (Fig. 5.4) (Ferrucci & Wittenberg, 1978). Parallel to the first needle positioned accurately within the pathological area, a second identical needle is placed up to five times within a minimum distance from the first needle, the last sample being taken through the first needle.

External guidance systems may facilitate the needle insertion parallel within the sagittal plane. This should allow precise positioning of the needle by means of a goniometer and a needle directing cuff (Fig. 5.5). By using the fixable needle directing plastic cuff, diversion from the sagittal axis is minimal, even when using fine needles. In addition, the indentation of the skin by the needle tip at the puncture site is avoided, and a more accurate depth position of the needle tip is thereby achieved.

With every CT-guided needle puncture, the correct three-dimensional position of the needle tip within the lesion should be verified by means of a *CT control scan*. Slight breathing movements during the exposure of the control scan with the needle positioned may lead to disturbing artefacts due to the needle metal (Fig. 5.6). A fast series of CT controlled scans by CT scanners with short exposure times from 2 - 5 secs and immediate image reconstruction are therefore of great importance.

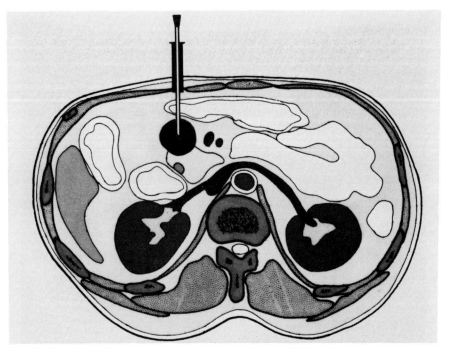

Fig. 5.3 Coaxial double needle puncture technique (Haaga & Alfidi, 1976).

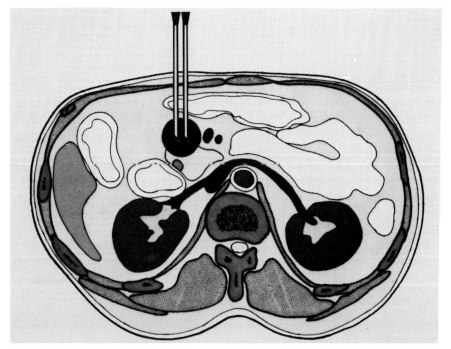

Fig. 5.4 Tandem needle technique (Ferrucci & Wittenberg, 1978).

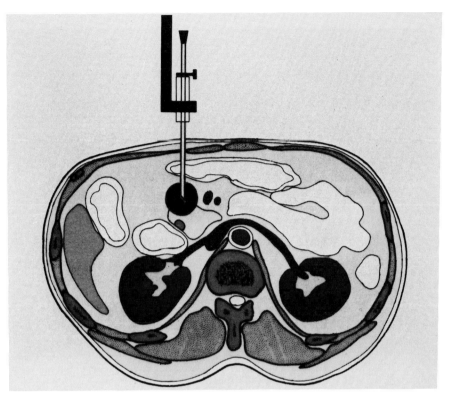

Fig. 5.5 External guidance system with needle directing cuff.

The *number of tissue samples* taken and the needle calibre are determining factors in guaranteeing successful results in aspiration biopsy. Three to five samples should be routinely taken to ensure positive cytological findings (Ferrucci et al, 1980). Successful cytological and histological diagnosis also depends on the careful *handling of the tissue specimens.* Due to insufficient fixation of the tissue samples the cells may become altered to a degree that cytological specification becomes impossible. Immediately following aspiration the biopsy material must be spread on a glass slide and then fixed, in order not to let the cellular tissue components dry out.

Complications following percutaneous aspiration biopsy are rare. Secondary peritonitis, pancreatitis or even fistulae have only been very rarely encountered (Ferrucci et al, 1980; Haaga et al, 1977). Small haematoma may occasionally occur. The risk of complication rises with the needle diameter. Major potential complications of percutaneous biopsies include bleeding as well as pneumothoraces. It should be routine to monitor the patient closely for some time after the biopsy. The risk of needle tract seeding and dissemination of malignant cells following fine-needle biopsies seems to be minimal (Engzell et al, 1971; Zajicek, 1974). However, a case of malignant seeding of the tract after thin-needle aspiration biopsy in carcinoma of the pancreas has been described recently (Ferrucci et al, 1979).

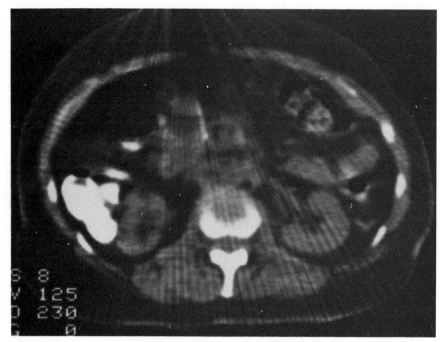

Fig. 5.6 CT control scan to verify the needle position within the mass lesion of the pancreatic head. Artefacts due to the metal needle and respiratory movements.

Severe bleeding disorders are *contra-indications* for needle biopsies. Echinococcal cysts are obviously also contra-indications for aspiration procedures.

Type and size of needles and catheters depend on the type of the aspiration procedure. For fine needle aspiration biopsy of the liver, pancreas, kidneys and lymphnodes, needles with a calibre of 0.65-0.9 mm external diameter (23-20 gauge) are preferable. Cytological specimens from small calibre needles are often non-conclusive in malignant lymphoma. Large calibre needles are, therefore, necessary, to obtain a tissue cylinder for histological investigation (Haaga, 1979). The same morphological problem applies for diffuse and focal liver lesions (Haaga & Vanek, 1979). Large bore 19-14 gauge needles and catheters 11.0-2.1 mm outer diameter are used for the diagnostic and therapeutic aspiration of cysts, abscesses or hematomas (Haaga et al, 1977).

Clinical indications

The clinical indications for CT-guided puncture have to be considered for each specific organ. They are mainly governed by the density, size and the topographic-anatomical localisation of the pathological lesions (Haaga & Reich, 1978).

Liver

Hepatic tumours, whether benign or malignant, primary or secondary, have similar tissue density values of 30-50 HU on CT and are, therefore, sometimes difficult to differentiate from the non-enhanced normal liver parenchyma with densities of 40-70 HU. There are no characteristic CT features of these lesions, and the lack of correlation with histological patterns is deceiving.

Guided needle biopsy is indicated to elucidate the cellular definition of focal metastatic lesions in the case of an unknown site of the primary tumor, to verify hepato-cellular carcinoma within a cirrhotic liver and to differentiate inflammatory from neoplastic focal lesions. In our case material 17 of 22 (75 per cent) liver lesions (usually metastases) were correctly identified.

Pancreas

Tumefaction and loss of peripancreatic and perivascular fat planes are important CT features indicating the presence of neoplasm. Chronic pancreatitis may, however, produce similar alterations depending on the degree of the inflammatory process. Guided fine needle biopsy should, therefore, be performed for conclusive cellular diagnosis whenever the slightest doubt about the presence of a malignant growth arises. In our case material malignant cells were identified by fine needle aspiration biopsy in 8 out of 15 pancreatic cancers.

Lymph nodes

Enlargement of lymph nodes demonstrated by CT is non-specific and may also be induced by reactive hyperplasia, or inflammation as well as malignant neoplasm. Consequently, CT-guided needle biopsy may be an important diagnostic tool for the conclusive etiological evaluation of the cellular pattern of retroperitoneal or intraperitoneal mass lesions.

Kidneys

Evaluation of renal masses and antegrade pyelography are the main indication for guided procedures of the kidneys. Guided cyst puncture and fluid aspiration is necessary in only about 2 per cent of cystic mass lesions, that is, when pain, haematuria or obstruction are present. Solid mass lesions which appear hypovascular on angio-CT give rise to particular diagnostic problems. The differentiation of inflammatory or other pseudo tumours, such as haematoma from partially necrotic neoplasms, may also become very difficult. The same applies to malignant mesenchymal neoplasms and papillary renal carcinoma. Guided fine needle biopsy may provide conclusive diagnostic results in such cases.

CT-guided antegrad pyelography and nephrostomy is done by percutaneous placement of catheters into the collecting system. Injection of contrast material provides a pyelogram demonstrating the point of obstruction. CT demonstration of the normal-sized renal pelvis makes its puncture possible even in a non-functioning kidney.

Abscess aspiration

CT is of particular diagnostic importance to demonstrate clinically suspected abscess formation. By obtaining a specimen by aspiration, bacteriological identification of the causative organisms permits selection of specific antibiotic therapy. Subpulmonary and subphrenic abscess locations are dramatically demonstrated when other methods, such as fluoroscopy and sonography have failed, because of the superposition of the bony structures of the thoracic cage.

Retroperitoneum

Neoplasms, abscesses, haematoma, lymphocele and urinoma within the retroperitoneum are ideally suited for CT guided aspirations. With the patients in a prone position, the lesion can be easily approached through a posterior entry point without damage to any vital structures. Local application of drugs for sympathetic blockade is selectively done under CT guidance.

Mediastinum, thoracic wall

Fine needle aspiration biopsy of mediastinal and thoracic wall mass lesions has been greatly facilitated by CT. The scan plane is set according to the findings on conventional radiographs. Bolus injection of contrast material improves delineation of the vascular structures prior to the selection of the entry point and the direction of the needle path.

Assessment of guidance methods

An essential difference between CT-controlled investigations and ultrasound or fluoroscopy guided aspiration techniques is the effort involved. Even with modern CT scanners several control investigations and manipulations of the needle within smaller lesions may be necessary and take more than 30 minutes, which increases the strain on the patient. Ultrasound affords an easier and faster result provided that a lesion is definable, because the desired biopsy material is obtained from a needle guided through the puncturing sound-emitting head, which in real time investigations is possible even under visual control. Further factors worth mentioning are the considerable difference in cost of the machines and the absence of radiation in the ultrasound method. Pulmonary lesions are well localised by fluoroscopy, and positive tissue sampling is possible with a high degree of accuracy. Based on these considerations, lesions easily demonstrated on ultrasonograms should be punctured by the ultrasound method. CT-guided puncture must be applied if compression of the skin due to the sound-emitting probe has to be avoided, as in the case of patients with post traumatic or post operative changes or with acute inflammatory diseases. Furthermore, the CT-guided puncture is a valid alternative method if the ultrasound is not successful, and is specifically so in adiposity, if there is superposition of gas or parts of the skeleton, and if the three-dimensional resolution necessary for small lesions can only be achieved by computed tomography. CT is advantageous with regard to the localisation of pathological lesions in hidden areas, such as the subphrenic and subpulmonary regions, as well as the mediastinum. For this reason our case material of ultrasound guided aspiration biopsies, comprising 240 consecutive cases, is about 5-fold that of the 48 CT-guided aspiration techniques.

Conclusions

Guided needle procedures are indicated in every mass lesion detected when the etiology is not clearly established. They should then be an integral part of the investigation procedure.

Aspiration biopsy can easily be performed and with great accuracy by ultrasound. Therefore, CT is indicated mainly when ultrasound guidance is not successful.

Needle procedures are elegant methods, with an accuracy rate of 60-80 per cent which lead directly to a conclusive cytopathological diagnosis. A positive result precludes further unnecessary investigations; a negative result is possibly non-diagnostic and has to be repeated. Through the use of guided needle techniques, exploratory operative interventions and operative drainage procedures can be avoided to the benefit of the patient.

References

Engzell U, Esposti P L, Rubio C 1971 Investigation on tumour spread in connection with aspiration biopsy. Acta radiologica 10: 385

Ferrucci J T, Wittenberg J 1978 CT biopsy of abdominal tumours: aids for lesion localisation. Radiology 129: 739

Ferrucci J T, Wittenberg J, Margolles M N, Carey R W 1979 Malignant seeding of the tract after thin-needle aspiration biopsy. Radiology 130: 345

Ferrucci J T, Wittenberg J, Mueller P R, Simeone J F, Harbni W P, Kirkpatrick R H, Taft P D 1980 Diagnosis of abdominal malignancy by radiologic fine-needle aspiration biopsy. American Journal of Roentgenology 134: 323

Haaga J R 1979 New techniques for CT-guided biopsies. American Journal of Roentgenology 133: 633

Haaga J R, Alfidi R J 1976 Precise biopsy localisation by computed tomography. Radiology 118: 603

Haaga J R, Reich N E 1978 Computed tomography of abdominal abnormalities. Mosby St Louis, p 315

Haaga J R, Vanek J 1979 Computed tomographic guided liver biopsy using the Menghini needle. Radiology 133: 405

Haaga J R, Alfidi R J, Havrilla T R, Coperman A M, Seidelmann F, Reich N, Weinstein A J, Meaney T F 1977 CT detection and aspiration of abdominal abscesses. American Journal of Roentgenology 128: 465

Stephenson T F, Mehnert P J, Marx A J, Boger J N, Roth-Moyo L, Balaji M R, Nadaraja N 1979 Evaluation of contrast markers for CT aspiration biopsy. American Journal of Roentgenology 133: 1097

Zajicek J 1974 Introduction to aspiration biopsy. Monogr. Clin. Cytol. 4: 1

6. Computed tomography in musculo-skeletal disease

I. ISHERWOOD

Introduction

The cross-sectional image provided by computed tomography (CT) of both appendicular and axial skeleton permits direct visualisation of trabecular and cortical bone whilst the sensitivity of CT to very small changes in X-ray attenuation occurring in soft tissues permits the visualisation of normal musculature and normal fat planes. The role of CT in the investigation of musculo-skeletal dirorders is currently under review (Berger & Kuhn, 1978; de Santos et al, 1978; McLeod et al, 1978; Schumaker et al, 1978; Wilson et al, 1978). The quantitative nature of the image provides a basis for measurement of bone mass and bone mineral at critical skeletal sites and of trabecular bone response to external stimuli.

Constraints

Despite the obvious advantages of a numerically-derived image and a uniformly thin section of tissue, there are a number of significant constraints inherent in the method.

1. Reproducibility

The thinner the CT section and the smaller the picture element (pixel) size, the greater the difficulty in obtaining precise positioning and accurate reproducibility in all spatial co-ordinates. The problem becomes most acute in those circumstances which require numerical data comparison over prolonged time intervals. No method yet proposed for achieving pixel reproducibility has proved entirely satisfactory in clinical practice without external fixation. External markers, together with 'scannogram' facilities provide the most useful approaches.

2. Boundary definition

An important feature in the analysis of bone and soft tissue disorders is the ability to define the edge of the anatomical or disease structure with accuracy. Many factors contribute to both systematic and random errors in linear and area measurement from CT images (Antoun et al, 1980).

3. Tissue characterisation

A unique advantage of CT is its ability in some circumstances to distinguish heterogeneity of tissue composition, particularly in those areas containing high (calcium) or low (fat) atomic number material. Despite this ability, however, precise histological characterisation is still not possible. A number of approaches towards tissue characterisation, including tomochemistry and an analysis of the distribution of attenuation values in both magnitude and space (Ritchings et al, 1980) have been employed. Detailed time sequence studies of intravenous contrast medium distribution also hold promise and are currently under investigation.

Bone

The success of CT in the analysis of disorders affecting bone relates to its ability to provide access to anatomical sites and physiological phenomena not easily imaged by other techniques. Some examples in the axial and appendicular skeleton will be discussed.

1. Axial skeleton

Pelvis and sacrum. As a result of difficulties in patient positioning or overlying bowel gas, conventional radiology may fail to detect significant areas of bone destruction in both primary and secondary malignant disease. The ischial spine (Fig. 6.1) and the body of the sacrum (Fig. 6.2) are sites particularly vulnerable to misinterpretation on plain films but readily displayed by CT.

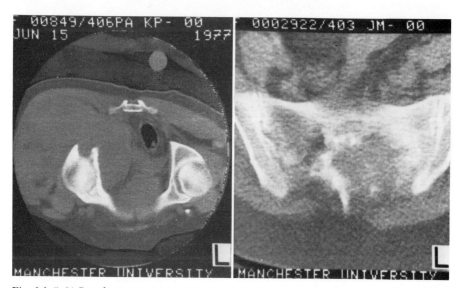

Fig. 6.1 (left) Paget's sarcoma left ischial spine. Patient prone. Bone erosion not visible on plain films due to rotation by soft tissue mass in buttock. Full extent of extra and intra pelvic soft tissue tumour with displacement of pelvic organs demonstrated by CT.

Fig. 6.2 (right) Carcinoma breast metastasis left sacrum. Plain film changes difficult to detect due to overlying bowel gas. Radio-isotope bone scan positive.

Spine. CT is not organ specific and axial sections of the spine therefore provide information about spinal morphology and pathology against a background of adjacent soft tissue and body cavity organs. Precise identification of the position and articular surface of apophyseal joints is possible, together with their relationship to the spinal canal and intervertebral foramina (Isherwood & Antoun, 1979). Spinal curvature may, however, result in significant variations in the anatomical features displayed on a single section of finite thickness. Caution must therefore be exercised in the interpretation of apparent bony abnormality displayed in single sections and also in the ready acceptance of linear or area measurement (Isherwood, Fawcitt et al, 1976).

The features most likely to influence clinical management in the initial radiological assessment of bony abnormalities of the spine are:

(i) *Extent of associated soft tissue abnormality.*

The thoraco-lumbar junction is frequently difficult to image by conventional radiology. An advantage of CT in this anatomical situation is its ability to display the extent of disease above and below the diaphragm and particularly in the retrocrural space (Fig. 6.3).

A   B

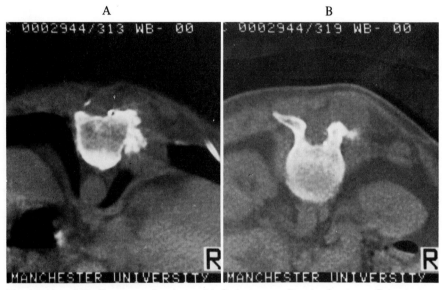

Fig. 6.3 (A and B) Recurrent chondroma L1. Patient prone. Post laminectomy. Subcutaneous nodule and retrocrural tumour extension demonstrated with associated calcium deposition. Extent of dural and neural involvement not possible without CT Myelography.

(ii) *Extent to which neural tissue in the spinal canal is involved.*

Identification of neural tissue involvement in the spinal canal is critical. Conventional CT is capable on occasion of identifying neural tissue in the cervical or lumbar spine where the CSF space is wide. In the thoracic spine, however, the CSF space is inconstant in its width and the dorsal cord anteriorly placed (Isherwood, Fawcitt et al, 1976). Variations in the factors affecting image quality have been explored to determine the optimal conditions for the demonstration of neural tissue within the spinal canal.

The factors affecting image quality are spatial resolution (picture element size), density discrimination (signal to noise), and radiation dose. These factors are inter-related and improvement in one cannot be made independently of the others (Pullan et al, 1976).

$$D \propto \frac{(S/N)^2}{R^3}$$

Spatial resolution: higher spatial resolution can be achieved and the dose penalty minimised by limiting the area of reconstruction (New, 1978). Higher resolution certainly provides added information in high density i.e. bony regions, and can be helpful in the identification of smaller bony structures (Lloyd et al, 1979). It does not necessarily, however, improve density discrimination.

Density discrimination: the ability to discriminate one soft tissue from another is improved by increasing the signal to noise ratio. At a fixed spatial resolution this may be achieved by increasing the photon flux, reducing the noise or increasing the density difference between adjacent tissues by the use of contrast media. In the spinal canal, water soluble contrast (Amipaque) can be introduced into the sub-arachnoid space (Isherwood et al, 1977) i.e. CT Myelography.

A combination of higher resolution and improved density discrimination without the use of contrast medium in the spinal canal has been proposed by Ethier et al (1979) employing a technique requiring repetitive high resolution limited area reconstruction sections to be added. Signal to noise ratios are thereby improved but local dose necessarily increased.

The hypothesis that this technique, giving higher resolution and lower noise levels, would allow consistent identification of the subarachnoid space has been tested in recent animal experiments (Isherwood et al, 1979). Using the pig as an experimental model it has been demonstrated that in situations where the sub-arachnoid space is narrow, i.e. less than 1-2 mm, even with added sections the subarachnoid space cannot be identified consistently without the use of sub-arachnoid contrast medium. CT myelography is therefore necessary for the full assessment of spinal canal involvement.

(iii) *The presence or absence of associated bony abnormalities.*

The vertebrae are the most frequent sites of skeletal metastases at autopsy in the common cancers (Jaffe 1958) and it is well known that a significant proportion of the vertebral body must be destroyed before the lesion is detectable by conventional radiology (Edelstyn et al, 1967). Whilst the role of radio-isotope bone scanning as a screening method is established in the study of metastatic bone disease, it is recognised that a number of non-malignant conditions may give rise to increased isotope activity. Degenerative arthritis of the axial synovial joints, apophyseal and costo-vertebral, are the commonest causes for such increased isotope uptake. A recent study by Best et al (1979) of 30 patients with proven carcinoma of the breast who had radio-isotope scans, radiographic skeletal surveys and CT scans suggested that in those patients CT could differentiate between metastatic disease and degnerative joint disease in the spine, even when the two were co-incident.

2. Appendicular skeleton (Destouet et al 1979; Heelan et al 1979; Hermann and Rose 1979; Weinberger and Levinsohm 1978; Weis et al 1978) *a. Trabecular bone space.* Differentiation of cortical and medullary bone is readily made in the cross-sectional image provided by CT and the response to tumour encroachment separately evaluated. Cortical erosion can be detected at an early stage in sites otherwise difficult to visualise (Fig. 6.4).

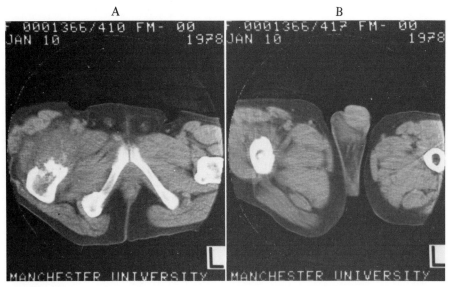

Fig. 6.4 (A and B) Chondrosarcoma right femoral neck. Anterior cortical destruction demonstrated with associated soft tissue mass. Increase in trabecular density due to associated enchondroma.

An accurate determination of the extension of tumour spread within the medullary cavity of long bones could be influential in the determination of amputation site. Increased attenuation values within the trabecular space have been attributed to direct tumour spread (Heelan et al, 1979) though inflammation, haemorrhage and simple reactive hyperplasia are known to give rise to similar changes at other sites. Experiments have been designed to assess the ability of CT to detect intramedullary tumour spread employing VX2 carcinoma in rabbit femora (Checkley et al, 1979). Reproducibility of CT section in these longitudinal studies has been achieved by the use of a specifically-designed animal sledge (Checkley & Best, 1979). Preliminary observations suggest that in the well-controlled experimental situation an increase in trabecular bone attenuation values following injection of VX2 carcinoma into the marrow cavity accurately reflects the histological appearances known to occur in the same situation. Nevertheless, other factors, e.g. saline injection in a control limb, can produce similar increases in attenuation values. The interpretation of changes in the trabecular space in the clinical situation should therefore be made with caution and the possibility of infection or associated haemorrhage considered.

b. Soft tissue extension. The ability of CT to discriminate soft tissue densities, particularly in the presence of well-defined fat planes, is well recognised and influences considerably the extent to which CT can affect clinical management.

Levine et al (1979) assessed the value of CT in 50 patients with musculo-skeletal tumours (Table 6.1) in terms of primary diagnosis, extent of tumour and influence on management. The presence of soft tissue extension significantly changed the level of influence of CT. A diagnostic imaging strategy for the investigation of musculo-skeletal tumours is proposed in Table 6.2.

Table 6.1 Musculo-skeletal tumours – value of CT in 50 patients, expressed as a percentage (after Levine et al, 1979 Radiology 131: 431–437)

	Bone only	Bone + Soft tissue	Soft tissue only	Total
Primary diagnosis	7.1	26.6	13.3	26
Tumour extent	28.5	86.6	66.6	54
Management planning	14.2	93.3	73.3	66

Table 6.2 Musculo-skeletal tumours – diagnostic strategy

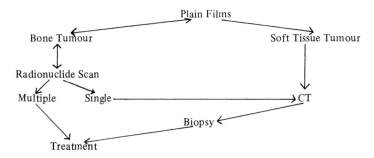

The role of CT in the primary investigation of bone tumours might be summarised thus:
1. The evaluation of equivocal radiographic changes.
2. The evaluation of the falsely positive isotope scan.
3. The identification and assessment of extent of associated soft tissue mass.
4. Cautious evaluation of medullary involvement.
5. Treatment planning and monitoring.

Role of CT in the assessment of pulmonary metastases

CT is a sensitive technique for the identification of non-calcified unsuspected nodules in the lung fields. Most metastatic disease affects the outer third of the lung fields and many metastases are subpleural or in the lung periphery. CT is therefore especially valuable in the detection of nodules in the costophrenic, retrosternal and retrocardiac spaces where conventional radiography is relatively insensitive (Fig. 6.5).

CT will detect more nodules than conventional radiology or whole lung tomography (Muhm et al 1978; Schaner et al 1978). Despite the improved sensitivity of CT, however, there is a significant lack of specificity and a proportion of nodules (up to 22 per cent) may go undetected. Many small nodules

42

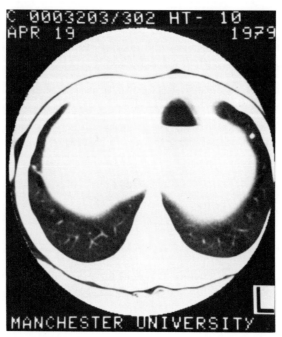

Fig. 6.5 Pulmonary metastases from pelvic round cell tumour in both costo-diaphragmatic sulci.

detected by CT are non-malignant. Up to 60 per cent of such lesions were recorded as benign granulomata in a carefully controlled study by Schaner et al (1978). Whilst this observation may represent a unique experience in the United States, it emphasises that CT does not at present replace conventional radiology in the assessment of pulmonary metastatic disease but only complements it.

Muscle

Most muscle groups related to the appendicular and axial skeleton are readily identified in the cross section. The number of muscles detected by CT increases with age and obesity as a result of increased deposition of fat in interstitial tissue. Changes in muscle bulk due to new growth are readily detected (Fig. 6.6). Variations due to differences in age and sex might be anticipated (Balcke et al, 1979). but are relatively minor. Neither intrinsic muscle disease nor neuro-muscular disease gives rise to specific CT appearances (Fig. 6.7). Deposition of fat and loss of muscle mass are features associated with those conditions leading to muscle atrophy. Changes in muscle density are observed less frequently and then related usually to ageing. The principal roles of CT in muscle disease are early detection of tumour in otherwise inaccessible sites (Fig. 6.8) and the subsequent monitoring of those processes together with the ability to delineate appropriate biopsy sites with precision.

CT angiography, i.e. CT during the first circulation following rapid high-dose intravenous injection of contrast medium, can be used to demonstrate variations

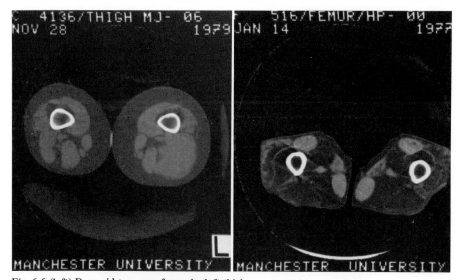

Fig. 6.6 (left) Desmoid tumour of muscle, left thigh.
Fig. 6.7 (right) Muscular dystrophy. Degeneration with fat deposition in muscles of both thighs.

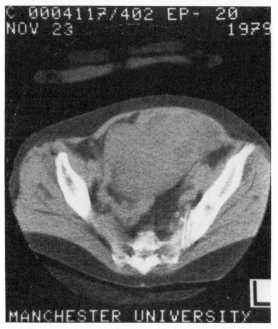

Fig. 6.8 Sarcoma arising in rectus abdominis muscle with intra-abdominal extension.

in vascularity particularly those associated with inflammation (Fig. 6.9). The role of CT angiography in tissue characterisation is currently under review. In summary,

CT in muscle disease has a high anatomical specificity and a low histological specificity.

Joint disease

CT of joint disease is most valuable in those situations where the partial volume effect is least obtrusive. In the smaller joints, very thin (2 mm) sections are necessary to overcome this effect. The reduction of section thickness results in further problems of reproducibility and increased noise.

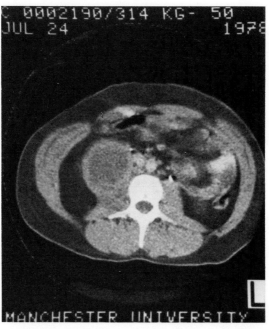

Fig. 6.9 Psoas abscess. CT angiography. Note contrast enhancement of abscess capsule.

In the pelvis, the transaxial section provided by CT is particularly appropriate for investigation of the hip and sacro-iliac joints (Lasda et al, 1978). The femoral head, anterior and posterior pillars of the acetabulum together with the long axis of the femoral neck, are demonstrable without the adoption of difficult and painful positions by the patient. The integrity of the joint in diseases affecting the femoral head is of obvious importance (Fig. 6.10).

A current review (Forbes et al) of adult female patients with congenital dislocation of the hip (Fig. 6.11) has indicated the value of CT in the assessment of acetabular capacity prior to femoral head replacement and has led to a critical review of the surgical approach to this group of patients.

In the assessment of femoral anteversion in infants, experimental studies (Witcombe) suggest that relatively small torsion effects produced by limb rotation can significantly affect angular measurement of the femoral neck.

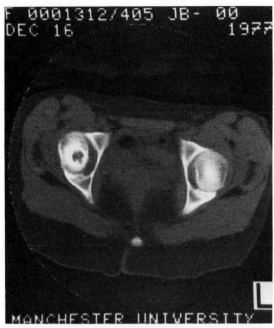

Fig. 6.10 Chondroblastoma right femoral head. Tri-foliate cavity with surrounding sclerosis. Note intact articular surface and normal joint cavity thus excluding villonodular synovitis.

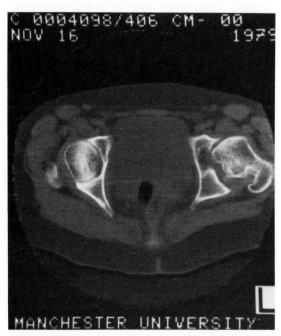

Fig. 6.11 Congenital dislocation left hip. Deformity of femoral head and acetabulum with anteversion of femoral neck.

46

Bone physiology

Bone mineral and bone mass measurements independent of subcutaneous fat and bony contour are possible by transaxial CT methods. A detailed review of these methods is beyond the scope of this review.

The accuracy and precision achieved in early studies of the forearm (Isherwood, Rutherford et al 1976) are difficult to reproduce in the axial skeleton and further studies are required to evaluate the influence of intramedullary fat on bone mineral measurement (Adams et al 1980). It must be recognised, however, that the mineral content of sample sites in the appendicular skeleton, even when obtained with accuracy and precision, may not necessarily reflect bone mineral content of those axial sites, e.g. vertebral body, with higher proportions of trabecular bone.

References

Adams J E, Isherwood I, Pullan B R, Ritchings R T, Adams P H 1980 The estimation of bone mass in vivo using CT scanning. European Seminar on Computed Tomography in Oncology, London

Antoun N M, Checkley D R, Isherwood I, Pullan B R, Ritchings R T 1980 Boundary definition by computed tomography. European Seminar on Computed Tomography in Oncology, London

Balcke J A, Termote J L, Palmers Y, Crolla D 1979 Computed tomography of the human skeletal muscular system. Neuroradiology 17: 127-136

Berger P E, Kuhn J P 1978 Computed tomography of tumours of the musculo-skeletal system in children. Radiology 127: 171-175

Best J J K, Forbes W StC, Adam N M, Isherwood I 1979 Computed tomographic scanning and radio-isotope bone scanning — a comparison. In: Gerhardt P, van Kaick G (ed) Total body computerised tomography Thieme, Stuttgart

Checkley D R, Best J J K 1979 A sledge device for the accurate movement of small animals in a computed tomographic scanner. Journal of Computer Assisted Tomography 3: 550-551

Checkley D R, Samuel W, Ritchings R T, Best J J K 1979 Computed tomography — bone tumour detection in the rabbit. International Conference on Information Processing in Medical Imaging, Paris

de Santos L A, Goldstein H M, Murray J A, Wallace S 1978 Computed tomography in evaluation of musculo-skeletal neoplasms. Radiology 128: 89-94

Destouet J M, Gilula L A, Murphy W A 1979 Computed tomography of long bone osteosarcoma. Radiology 131: 439-445

Edelstyn G A, Gillespie P J, Grebbell F S 1967 The radiological demonstration of osseous metastases — experimental observations. Clinical Radiology 18: 158-162

Ethier R, King D G, Melancon D, Belanger G, Taylor S, Thompson C 1979 Development of high resolution computed tomography of the spinal cord. Journal of Computer Assisted Tomography 3: 433-438

Forbes W StC, Isherwood I, Hardings K Computed tomography in adult congenital dislocation of the hip (in preparation)

Heelan R T, Watson R C, Smith J 1979 Computed tomography of lower extremity tumours. American Journal of Roentgenology 132: 933-937

Hermann G, Rose J S 1979 Computed tomography in bone and soft tissue pathology of the extremities. Journal of Computer Assisted Tomography 3: 58–66

Isherwood I, Fawcitt R A, Forbes W StC, Nettle J R L, Pullan B R 1977 Computed tomography scanning in the assessment of lumbar spine problems. In: Jayson M I V (ed) The lumbar spine and back pain. Pitman Medical, London

Isherwood I, Antoun N M, Checkley D R, Dovas T 1979 Experience with high resolution scanning of the spine. Journal of Computer Assisted Tomography 3: 566-567

Isherwood I, Rutherford R A, Pullan B R, Adams P H 1976 Bone mineral estimation by computer assisted transverse axial tomography. Lancet 2: 712-715

Isherwood I, Fawcitt R A, Forbes W StC, Nettle J R L, Pullan B R 1977 Computed tomography of the spinal canal using Metrizamide. Acta radiologica Supplement 355: 299

Isherwood I, Fawcitt R A, Nettle J R L, Spencer J W, Pullan B R 1976 Computed tomography of the spine. In: du Boulay G H, Moseley I F (ed) Computerised axial tomography in clinical practice. Soringer-Verlag, Berlin p 322-335

Jaffe H L 1958 Tumours, tumomas – conditions of the bones and joints. Lea & Feloger, Philadelphia

Lasda N A, Levinsohn E M, Yuan H A, Bumnell W P 1978 Computerised tomography in disorders of the hip. Journal of Bone and Joint Surgery 60A: 1099-1102

Levine E, Lee K R, Neff J R, Malad N F, Robinson R G, Preston D F 1979 Comparison of computed tomography and other imaging modalities in the evaluation of musculo-skeletal tumours. Radiology 131: 431-437

Lloyd G A S, du Boulay G H, Phelps P D, Pullicino P 1979 The demonstration of the auditory ossicles by high resolution computed tomography. Neuroradiology 18: 242-248

McLeod R A, Stephens D H, Boabout J W, Sheedy P F, Hattery R R 1978 Computed tomography of the skeletal system. Seminars in Roentgenology 13: 235-247

Muhm J R, Brown L R, Crowe J K, Sheedy P F, Hattery R R, Stephens D H 1978 Comparison of whole lung tomography and computed tomography for detecting pulmonary nodules. American Journal of Roentgenology 131: 981-984

New P F J 1978 CT5005 (EMI Medical Systems) High resolution scanning. Neuroradiology 16: 530-531

Pullan B R, Rutherford R A, Isherwood I 1976 Computerised transaxial tomography. In: Hay G A (ed) Medical images – formation, perception and measurement. Wiley, Bristol p 20

Ritchings R T, Isherwood I, Pullan B R 1980 Tissue characterisation – does it work? European Symposium on Computer Assisted Tomography (2)

Schaner E G, Chang A E, Doppman J L, Conkle D M, Flye M W, Rosenberg S A 1978 Comparison of computed and conventional whole lung tomography in detecting pulmonary nodules – a prospective radiologic-pathologic study. American Journal of Roentgenology 131: 51-54

Schumaker T M, Genant H K, Korobkin M, Bovill E G 1978 Computed tomography – its use in space occupying lesions of the musculo-skeletal system. Journal of Bone and Joint Surgery 60A: 600-607

Weinberger G, Levinsohm E M 1978 Computed tomography in the evaluation of sarcomatous tumours of the thigh. American Journal of Roentgenology 130: 115-118

Weis L, Heelan R T, Watson R C 1978 Computed tomography of orthopaedic tumours of the pelvis and lower extremities. Clinical Orthopaedics and Related Research 130: 254-259

Wilson J S, Korobkin M, Genant H K, Bovill E G 1978 Computed tomography in musculo-skeletal disorders. American Journal of Roentgenology 131: 55-61

Witcombe J B Personal communication

7. The capabilities and limitations of CT in paediatric oncology

KAREN DAMGAARD-PEDERSEN

Multiple diagnostic procedures are performed in the initial investigation of paediatric patients with malignant diseases to obtain as much information as possible about the type, site, and extent of tumour spread. The staging procedures are of vital importance in the evaluation of the prognosis of the child and in the choice of therapeutic approach, between surgery, radiation and/or chemotherapy. Furthermore, the long term follow up of these patients includes further examinations during and after the treatment to estimate therapeutic response.

The following report deals with our experience with CT whole-body scanning in the diagnosis, staging and follow up of 115 children with various types of extracranial malignancy (Table 7.1). The patient age ranged from 5 days to 15 years with a median age of approximately 4 years. The equipment used is an EMI 5005 General Purpose Scanner with a scan time of 18 seconds.

Table 7.1 Number of examinations performed in 115 children with malignant diseases. Column I illustrates the number of patients and examinations where CT was performed in the primary investigation and staging, and column II shows the number of scannings performed in the total number of patients examined in the follow up period.

Type of malignancy	No. of patients	Primary tumour invest. No. of scannings I	Follow up No. of scannings II	Total No. of scannings
Wilms' tumour	28	11	63	74
Neuroblastoma	25	13	26	39
Malignant lymphoma	10	8	19	27
Teratoma	8	6	24	30
Rhabdomyosarcoma	6	2	13	17
Leukemia	34	34	4	38
Miscellanous	4	4	23	27
Total	115	78	172	250

Patient Preparation

Sedation and anaesthesia

Co-operation can only be obtained in a limited number of the patients and sedation is necessary in children less than six years. The drug of choice is Vallergan[R] (Alimemazin) in a dose of 3mg/kg orally 2 - 3 hours before the examination.

General anaesthesia has been used in approximately 20 per cent of the examinations, most often in children 2–3 years old, the most difficult age to handle. The advantage of general anaesthesia is high quality scans without motion artefacts. But disadvantages exist: an oral contrast medium cannot be given and pseudotumour formation of the intestines might handicap the interpretation of the abdominal scans. Secondly, but not less important: the anaesthesia induces high-absorptive confluent areas in the lower dorsal part of the lungs. The abnormalities have been observed in 80 per cent of the pulmonary scans in the children anaesthetised with Halothane. These anaesthesia-induced alterations are without clinical significance, but it is important not to misinterpret these high absorptive areas as pathological changes and to realise, that epidiaphragmatic metastases can be missed in patients with pronounced changes. For this reason we always try to perform pulmonary CT using sedation only, since sedation does not affect the appearance of the lung parenchyma.

Contrast agents

Pseudotumourformation from the intestines is a general problem in the interpretation of the abdominal scans, unless the intestines are opacified. We use a 2 per cent solution of Telebrix[R] 380 mg/ml (Joxitalamate) an ideal tasteless medium, generally accepted by the children. This solution is given to all the children 2 hours and half an hour before the examination. Apart from preventing pseudo tumour formation, the opacified intestines improve the delineation of the abdominal organs and the pre- and paravertebral structures, which are generally ill-defined due to the relative paucity of retroperitoneal fat. When parenchymal enhancement of the liver and the kidneys is required, we use 60 per cent Urografin (megmonine/Sodium diatrizoate) in a dose of 1.5 ml/kg as bolus injection, intravenously.

Antiperistaltics

In our experience, using an 18 second scanner, it is essential to prevent disturbing artefacts from intestinal movements. Acceptable paralysis is generally obtained with Buscopan[R] (Hyoscine-N-Butylbromide) in a dose of 1mg/kg intramuscularly immediately before the examination. No adverse reactions to Buscopan have been noticed in our patients.

Primary tumour investigation

Wilms' tumour

Intravenous urography is the important initial investigation to be performed in patients suspected of Wilms' tumour, but CT should be applied as an important additional non-invasive examination in all cases with abnormal findings to further evaluate the nature and extent of the lesion. CT is able to differentiate between a solid renal tumour and benign cystic lesions, and to display the underlying cause of a urographic non-functioning kidney.

The CT appearance of a Wilms' tumour is typically a relatively low attenuation slightly inhomogeneous tumour (Fig. 7.1). In eleven patients examined the tumour

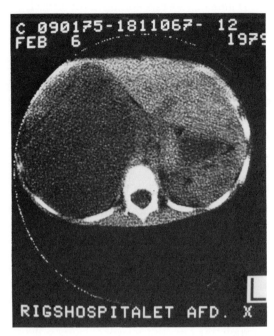

Fig. 7.1 A large right-sided Wilms' tumour in a 4-year-old boy. The tumour is well-delineated and demarcated from the normal, but displaced liver. There is no affection of the caval vein and the aorta.

was well-delineated, uncalcified and confined to the one side of the abdomen. Small tumours can be separated from the surrounding parenchyma following contrast enhancement (Fig. 7.2), whereas large tumours totally obliterate the renal space and normal parenchyma cannot be identified. Perirenal bleeding due to tumour induced rupture of the capsule was observed in one case. The haematoma simulated solid tumour formation, but the perirenal collection was identified following contrast enhancement of the renal parenchyma (Fig. 7.3). CT is not able to differentiate between Wilms' tumour and its variants, including the benign mesoblastic nephroma. The important aspect of CT in this part of the initial investigation is to estimate the true extent of the tumour and to predict the operability by evaluating involvement of the perivascular structures. A well-delineated caval vein and aorta is a reliable sign of resectability, but it is necessary to stress that intravascular tumour formation and capsule involvement (Green & Jaffe, 1978 a) has not so far been demonstrated in our patients.

Neuroblastoma

This most common solid extracranial malignant tumour can be situated throughout the area of the sympathetic chain and in the adrenal glands (Koop & Johnson, 1971). Tumours of the neck have not been seen in our material, which includes tumours in the mediastinum, the retroperitoneal space and the adrenals. In the chest small tumours appear as paravertebral lesions, well-delineated from the lung

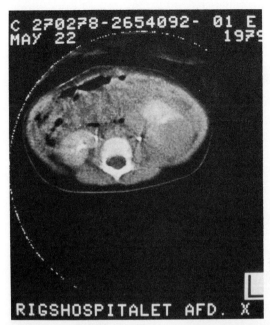

Fig. 7.2 A 14-month-old girl with a Wilms' tumour in the dorso-lateral part of the left kidney. The normal contrast enhanced parenchyma is displaced anteriorly.

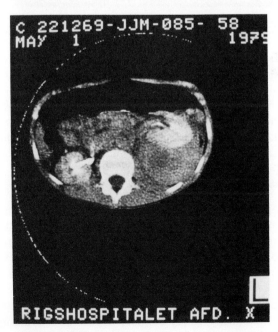

Fig. 7.3 A large retrorenal subcapsular haemorrhage in a 9-year-old boy with a small Wilms' tumour in the upper pole of the left kidney.

parenchyma, whereas large tumours displace and obliterate the mediastinal structures and expand into the chest cavity. In the same way the abdominal neuroblastomas most often obliterate the retroperitoneal space, surround the vessels and displace the neighbouring organs (Berger et al, 1978) (Fig. 7.4).

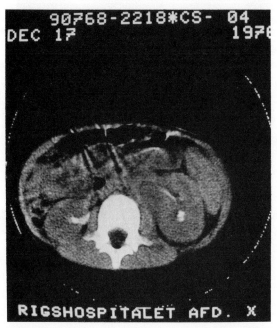

Fig. 7.4 A 9-year-old girl with a left-sided retroperitoneal neuroblastoma. The cystic tumour displaces the kidney laterally and obliterates the fat tissue planes of the adjacent structures.

Well-delineated adrenal lesions were found by CT in two of the 13 patients examined as part of the primary investigation. The CT appearance varies with the size of the tumour, but typically the tumour has a high density with minor or major cystic areas. Calcifications have been found in more than half of our patients examined. Important differential diagnoses with CT are teratomas and, when abdominally situated, large nephroblastomas, but a significant increase of Vanillin Mandelic Acid (VMA) finally establishes the diagnosis.

Malignant lymphoma/lymphosarcoma

Bipedal lymphography is often difficult to perform in children, and CT offers an important non-invasive method in the evaluation of the abdominal lymph nodes. As the retroperitoneal structures are often ill-defined, opacification of the intestines is mandatory to avoid 'pseudolymphomaformation' from the intestinal loops. The normal abdominal lymph nodes are generally not visible in small children, and a well-delineated pre- and para-aortic area with preserved fat tissue plans around the caval vein and the aorta excludes, in most cases, lymphomatous involvement of the nodes, Abnormally enlarged nodes appear as high-absorptive lobulated areas, which obliterates the perivascular structures and displaces the intestines anteriorly and laterally. The limitations of CT in the evaluation of the lymph nodes are, that abnormalities can only be identified due to enlargement of the nodes, whereas structural changes cannot be seen (Harell et al, 1977).

Teratomas

A preoperative diagnosis of these tumours can often be made by CT due to the various tissue elements identified as soft tissue, fat and calcifications (Fig. 7.5).

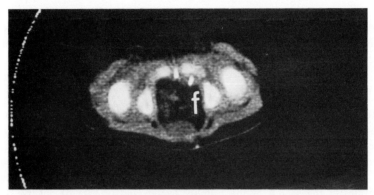

Fig. 7.5 A benign pelvic teratoma in a 2-month-old girl. The tumour contains large amounts of fat (f). The urethra and the rectum are filled with contrast, the latter displaced anteriorly by the tumour.

Mediastinal or abdominal homogeneous teratomas with scattered calcification cannot be differentiated from neuroblastomas (Fig. 7.6). As in other types of

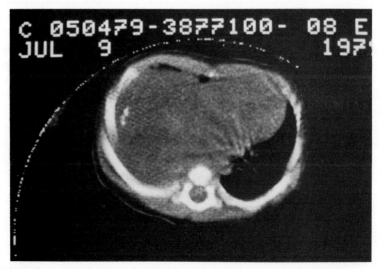

Fig. 7.6 A 3-month-old boy with a large malignant teratoma containing minor cystic areas and calcifications. The tumour arose from the right diaphragm and obliterated almost the entire right chest cavity.

tumours CT is important in the evaluation of the size and resectability, whereas malignancy can only be diagnosed preoperatively when signs of metastases are revealed, either nodal or pulmonary.

Rhabdomyosarcoma

Only a few patients with this rare malignancy have been evaluated primarily or during therapy by CT. The tumours have been localised to the chestwall, to the upper abdomen and the uro-genital area. CT is an important supplement to conventional radiological investigations in visualising involvement of the surrounding structures, but no specific CT appearance of the tumour can be described. As nodal metastasis are common (Green & Jaffe, 1978b) the area of the primary and secondary lymph drainage should always be included in the scanning.

Miscellanous

A limited number of paediatric patients offer a specific problem in the primary oncological investigation, as they present with metastases and clinical investigations and conventional radiologic examinations fail to reveal a primary tumour. CT has been used in four patients of this kind, but without success. In these patients it can be a great help to perform scintigraphic examinations with Gallium and Technetium in the search of the primary lesion, and in case of positive findings CT should be applied in the area of abnormal accumulation to evaluate the nature and extent of the focus (Damgaard-Pedersen et al, 1979).

Leukaemia

In our opinion, CT body scanning has so far no significant clinical importance in this field of childhood malignancy. This opinion is based on the investigation with CT in more than thirty patients, most of whom had an acute lymphoblastic leukaemia. CT has been performed at the time of diagnosis or at the time of a haematological or localised relapse. Enlargement of the liver and spleen was found in a number of the patients which was consistent with the clinical findings. The attenuation numbers of the enlarged liver and spleen did not differ from those in normal organs.

A few exceptions must be made to this general statement of the value of CT in children with leukaemia. In patients with mediastinal involvement at the time of presentation, CT should be used to examine the subdiaphragmatic lymph nodes. Secondly, it is obvious that when these children need further investigation in relation to complications of their malignancy or the subsequent therapy, CT can be used as a non-invasive method for the diagnosis of abscesses or intra-abdominal haematomas (Boldt & Reilly, 1977).

Staging

Anatomical staging of the tumour

Numerous systems are used in staging of the various malignant tumours in childhood. Generally these criteria include a patho-anatomical staging of the extent and invasiveness of the primary tumour and a clinical staging of the patients concerning metastatic disease. The efficacy of CT in the anatomical staging or preoperative evaluation of localised disease and resectability has been described under the various types of tumour examined. In the following section the capabilities and limitations of CT in clinical staging will be discussed concerning the detection of secondary spread to the lungs, liver and bones. The aspects of CT in the evaluation of lymph nodes are discussed in connection with malignant lymphoma.

Metastases

The lungs. CT is the most sensitive method in the evaluation of pulmonary metastases (Muhm et al, 1977). The detectable size is about 3 — 5 mm. Besides parenchymal metastases, CT is able to reveal very small pleural metastases and minor pleural effusions, undetectable in conventional films. Abnormal lymph nodes in the paratracheal area or the pulmonary hilus are more difficult to diagnose with CT, the detectable critical size being approximately 1 — 2 cm. Due to the high sensitivity of CT in the detection of metastases, the lungs are always included when CT scanning is performed in a primary tumour investigation. Parenchymal metastases have been revealed in patients with Wilms' tumours and teratomas, and pleural deposits and effusions in more patients with neuroblastoma and malignant lymphoma. As pulmonary CT cannot be performed in all patients during therapy and follow up due to a restricted capacity, it is our policy to use CT of the lungs supplementary to conventional examinations, when the chest film indicates further investigation.

The liver. Metastases can be revealed, when large enough. A critical detectable size cannot be estimated, as large superficial metastases can be overlooked and small well-delineated deepseated deposits can be detected, depending on the differences in absorption coefficients between the normal parenchyma and the focal lesion. Furthermore, it is necessary to emphasize, that a reliable evaluation of the liver depends totally on the quality of the examination. Motion-artefacts, due to patient anxiety and respiration together with streaks from intestinal gas influence liver visualisation, and indeed these factors are the greatest limitations of CT in clinical staging. As we do not routinely use intravenous contrast medium in the evaluation of the liver, it is not possible to estimate whether contrast enhancement improves the diagnostic sensivity of CT in these patients, but we know, that any injection disturbs the children with subsequent further degrading of the quality of the scans.

The truncal skeleton. The skeleton included in the body scan is always evaluated with window-settings for bone visualisation in the search for osseous lesions. Normally, the upper part of the dorsal spine is difficult to display optimally due to streaking artefacts from air in the trachea. The spine caudal to the tracheal bifurcation and the pelvic bones are well visualised and structural changes can be identified. Sclerotic metastasis can be revealed even when very small (Fig. 7.7) whereas minor lytic destructions are more difficult to detect. Furthermore, it is important to stress, that metastatic vertebral destruction and collapse can be overlooked due to the transverse display of the anatomy as observed in two patients in our material. CT can add important information concerning osseous lesions in

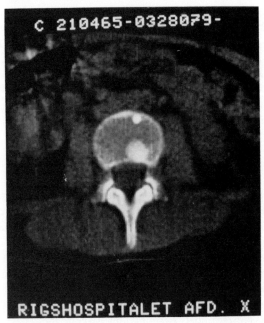

Fig. 7.7 Sclerotic metastases in a lumbar vertebra in a 13-year-old girl with an anaplastic malignant tumour of unknown origin.

the truncal skeleton, but cannot replace the skeleton radiographic survey and bone scintigraphy in the staging of these patients.

CT in the management and follow up of treated malignancy

In this aspect of paediatric oncology, CT first of all serves as an excellent method for radiation therapy field planning, as the technique is able to display the true extent of a tumour in a three dimensional manner. Furthermore, therapeutic response is well estimated by CT enabling appropriate alteration of the field during the treatment. When radiation and/or chemotherapy has been applied as a pre-operative treatment of the patient, CT can be used in the estimation of resectability of the tumour (Damgaard-Pedersen et al, 1978; Bullimore et al, 1979). Finally, CT serves as an important non-invasive method in the evaluation of local recurrence or progression of a tumour remnant in areas previously difficult to evaluate, especially in the retroperitoneal space (Fig. 7.8) and the pelvis.

It is obvious that CT should be performed when there is clinical suspicion of relapse or progression, but the question exists, whether CT should be included in the general survey of patients during the long term follow up? This question is of special interest in paediatric patients, in whom it is most important to obtain as much information as possible in a non-invasive harmless fashion.

During a three-year-period we have performed CT in the concurrent control of patients, when clinical conditions indicated further investigations as well as in patients at fixed intervals during the treatment and follow up period. An analysis

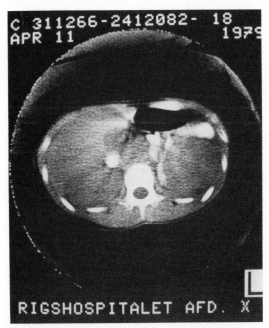

Fig. 7.8 A local recurrence in a 13-year-old girl, in whom a left nephrectomy was performed three years previously because of a large Wilms' tumour. Note the displacement of the opacified intestines.

of all these examinations (Table 7.1) showed, than when CT revealed a local recurrence, progression or metastases, the examinations had in most cases been dictated by other investigations or clinical findings. CT did not reveal unexpected findings in patients, who were clinically in complete remission. It is therefore our opinion, that CT, at least when the capacity is restricted, should not be used in the general survey of patients treated for a low stage tumour, when they are in clinical remission. However, CT should be performed in patients with high risk of relapse or tumour-remnants, even when clinical investigations do not give suspicion of progression. These considerations are so far necessary, as there is still a question as to how to use effectively and to best advantage, the capacity of the existing equipment.

Conclusion

When the role of CT in paediatric oncology is generally considered, it is our experience that CT offers a unique method in the evaluation of the nature, site and extent of a space-occupying lesion. Furthermore, CT provides important additional information in the clinical staging of the patients and during the long term follow up, when local recurrence or progression is suspected. The described existing limitations are commonly related to the quality of the scans. It is most likely that the diagnostic ability of CT in this category of patients will be further improved with the development of high resolution systems with considerable reduced scan time and slice thickness.

58

References

Berger P E, Kuhn J P, Munschauer R W 1978 Computed tomography and ultrasound in the diagnosis and management of neuroblastoma. Radiology 128: 663–667

Boldt D W, Reilly B J 1977 Computed tomography of abdominal mass lesions in children. Radiology 124: 371–378

Bullimore J A, Jones B, Davies E R, Shandell Y 1979 Computed tomography as an aid to staging and management of childhood malignancy. Xtract 7: 24–30

Damgaard-Pedersen K, Jensen J, Herts H 1978 CT whole-body scanning in paediatric radiology. Paediatric Radiology 6: 222–229

Damgaard-Pedersen K, Edeling C J, Hertz H 1979 CT whole-body scanning and scintigraphy in children with malignant tumours. Paediatric Radiology 8: 103–107

Green D M, Jaffe N 1978a Wilms' tumour-model of a curable paediatric malignant solid tumour. Cancer Treatment Reviews 5: 143–172

Green D M, Jaffe N 1978b Progress and controversy in the treatment of childhood rhabdomyosarcoma. Cancer Treatment Reviews 5: 7–27

Harell G S, Breiman R S, Glatstein E J, Marshall W H, Castellino R A 1977 Computed tomography of the abdomen in the malignant lymphomas. Radiologic Clinics of North America XV(3): 391–400

Koop C E, Johnson D G 1971 Neuroblastoma: an assessment of therapy in reference to staging. Journal of Paediatric Surgery 6(5): 595–600

Muhm I R, Brown L R, Crowe J K 1977 Detection of pulmonary nodules by computed tomography. American Journal of Roentgenology 128: 267–278

8. Do we need CT for the management of lymphomas?

JONATHAN BEST and GEORGE BLACKLEDGE

Introduction

In a patient with cancer, staging is performed to guide selection of therapy and to identify the parameters of disease that can be followed to assess the efficacy of treatment. Development of a standardised staging classification for disease provides a common system for describing the extent and involvement and enabling comparisons and where appropriate, pooling observations. This collected experience serves as a yardstick against which both the prognosis of an individual patient and the results of therapeutic trials can be measured.

Patients with Hodgkin's disease are likely to have apparent localised disease after extensive staging procedures and an appreciable proportion may have limited disease usually above the diaphragm which may be adequately treated by radio-therapy. The very much worse prognosis of patients inadequately treated, however, has led to the use of a staging laparotomy and splenectomy as part of the initial assessment.

At the First European Seminar in Computed Tomography in 1976, a pilot study of the role of CT as a non-invasive staging and monitoring procedure was reported (Best & Isherwood, 1977). It will be the purpose of this paper to report on this experience with particular reference to the abdominal staging of patients with Hodgkin's disease.

Materials and methods

A total of 176 patients presenting for the first time with Hodgkin's disease and entered into the Manchester Lymphoma Group studies of HD were referred between July 1976 and October 1979, from the Christie Hospital to the Department of Diagnostic Radiology, University of Manchester, for CT scans of the abdomen (Best et al, 1978; Blackledge et al, 1980). The diagnosis was made on a lymph node biopsy and the histology classified using the Rye nomenclature for Hodgkin's disease (Lukes & Butler, 1966). At presentation when the disease had been confirmed by histology, each patient was staged as accurately as possible using the Ann Arbor classification (Carbone et al, 1971).

Bi-pedal lymphography was performed in those patients who were Stage I, II or IIA and who had no medical contra-indication to the procedure. The total dose of Lipiodol did not exceed 14 ml. Criteria for nodal involvement were (a) nodal enlargement with separation of contrast-filling sinuses ('foamy' appearance);

(b) filling defects other than at the node hilum (seen on at least two different projections); (c) absence of node filling, often associated with abnormal collateral vessels. Additional signs were (d) filling of nodes at abnormal sites and (e) displacement of nodes from the vertebral column.

Laparotomy was performed in those patients medically suitable with clinical stages IA, IB, IIA, IIB and IIIA. The spleen and splenic hilar lymph nodes were removed. Biopsy specimens were taken from the nodes in the iliac and para-aortic groups and also from nodes that are not usually shown on a lymphogram including those in the coeliac axis, mesentery and omentum. Biopsy sites were marked with tantalum clips. Wedge and needle biopsies of the liver were performed. A fuller account of the staging procedures is given elsewhere (Blackledge et al, 1980).

All patients were scanned with an EMI CT 5000 Whole Body Scanner, updated in July 1977 to the EMI CT 5005. Patients were prepared before the examination with a bulk laxative for two days (Isogel, 10 ml b.d.) and 30 minutes before scanning were given 250 ml of Gastrografin diluted to 5 per cent v/v orally. Immediately prior to the scan, the bowel was paralysed by an injection of Propantheline, 100 mg i.m. All patients were scanned supine, holding their breath in inspiration. The patients were scanned at 140 kVp and 28 mA and with a 20 second scan time.

Patients with Hodgkin's disease were scanned from the level of the xiphisternum caudally using 13 mm collimation. The first 8 cm were scanned at 1 cm intervals and then scans were performed at 2 cm intervals to the level of the superior anterior iliac spines. Scanning was continued caudally if there was a specific reason for examining below that level, e.g. the patient presenting with large nodes in the groin.

The maximum skin entry dose was 5.3 rads (Isherwood, 1978).

Scan pictures were regarded as showing involvement by lymphoma if lymph node enlargement was demonstrated, i.e. if lymph nodes were greater than 1.5 cm in diameter. Lymph nodes smaller than 1.5 cm in diameter in certain areas carried a high index of suspicion. These areas were the retrocrural space and the left para-aortic region. The liver was considered enlarged if it was seen on the scan pictures below the ribs in the mid-axillary line. The spleen was considered enlarged if it was seen on scan pictures below the ribs. Extra-nodal involvement was diagnosed if the normal contour or architecture of the abdominal organs was distorted. Interpretation of the scan picture was based on morphological criteria. Diagnosis of osseous involvement required either loss of the normal bony outlines with associated loss of fascial planes implying adjacent soft tissue infiltration or increased attenuation above normal values for bone.

Intravenous contrast enhancement was employed only in the following circumstances:

1. Low attenuation areas in the liver and spleen, such areas were considered to be abnormal if they did not enhance after intravenous contrast.

2. Suspicion of renal involvement and ureteric obstruction.

Results

The results of CT of the abdomen in staging Hodgkin's disease represent an updating of a continuous trial whose interim results previously have been reported

(Best et al, 1978; Crowther et al, 1979; Blackledge et al, 1980). There were 176 patients, the distribution of histology and final pathological staging is shown in Table 8.1. 105 patients had a laparotomy performed. The results of CT compared with laparotomy are shown in Table 8.2, and the correlation with the sites of

Table 8.1 Stage and pathology

Pathology	Stage				
	I	II	III	IV	Total
LP	18	8	11	3	40
NS	9	17	8	10	44
MC	18	16	26	29	89
LD	0	0	0	3	3
Total	45	41	45	45	176

LP = lymphocyte predominant

NS = nodular sclerosing

MC = mixed cellularity

LD = lymphocyte depleted

Table 8.2 Results of CT compared with laparotomy in 105 patients with Hodgkin's disease

Laparotomy Results	No.	CT -ve	CT +ve	CT false +ve
Negative laparotomy	63	58	5	5
Positive laparotomy	42	31*	11	1

*includes 30 +ve spleens

involvement as demonstrated by CT compared with the disease found at laparotomy as shown in Table 8.3. In 42 patients evidence of Hodgkin's disease

Table 8.3 CT compared with assessment at laparotomy by site of involvement in 105 patients with Hodgkin's disease

Confirmed site of involvement	No. +ve at lap	CT +ve	CT false +ve
Spleen	36	6	1
Liver	11	5	3
Coeliac	7	2	0
Splenic hilum	4	2	0
Mesenteric	3	0	1
Para-aortic	10	4	2
Iliac	3	1	0

was found at operation. CT did not detect disease in 31 of the 42 positive cases and in 30 of these 31 positive patients, the spleen was involved by Hodgkin's disease. 44 of the patients were investigated by CT, lymphography and laparotomy and comparative results are shown in Table 8.4. A further 16 patients had CT and lymphography alone and the comparative results of the total group of 60 patients who had both CT and lymphography are shown in Table 8.5. When compared with

Table 8.4 Results of laparotomy compared with CT and lymphography in assessing nodal involvement in 44 patients with Hodgkin's disease

Laparotomy Results	No.	CT-ve	CT+ve	CT false+ve	L-ve	L+ve	L false+ve
Lap. -ve	28	27	1	1	28	0	0
Lap. +ve	16	10	6	0	14	3	1

Table 8.5 Comparison of CT and lymphography in 60 patients with untreated Hodgkin's disease

	No.	Total CT +ve	CT +ve in lymphogram area	CT -ve	CT +ve outside lymphogram area
Lymphogram -ve	51	7	3	44	4
Lymphogram +ve	9	9	9	0	6

laparotomy, the number of times CT and lymphography were reported as false-positive or negative were similar. If the total number of patients who had lymphography is compared with CT (Table 8.5), CT compares favourably with lymphography. In 10 out of 60 cases, CT showed additional disease beyond the area which was examined by lymphography — that is the iliac and lower and mid para-aortic lymph nodes. In 3 cases where the lymphogram was normal, CT detected disease in the lymphographic area. In two of these cases, laparotomy was performed and this confirmed the disease histologically.

Discussion

The primary purpose of this study was to assess whether CT might replace laparotomy which is a major investigative procedure with a small but definite morbidity and with a risk of mortality, albeit very small (Kawarada et al, 1976). In the study CT has not been used as a diagnostic procedure. In all cases the diagnosis and the histological sub-type of the patient had been known before CT examination was performed. This has allowed the adoption of laxer criteria in interpretation of the examination with a higher index of suspicion than might have been used in a screening context.

When compared with laparotomy, the results of CT are disappointing (Table 8.2 and 8.3). This refers especially to the detection of disease in the spleen where only 6 of 36 diseased spleens were detected. In the 31 cases where CT was negative and laparotomy detected disease, 30 spleens were involved by Hodgkin's disease. The 6 spleens that were regarded as abnormal by CT were all enlarged sufficiently to be seen below the costal margin.

If the accuracy of CT compared with laparotomy is assessed in terms of a decision matrix (Table 8.6) the specificity is seen to be 92 per cent and the

Table 8.6 CT compared with laparotomy 105 patients

	Disease +ve	Disease -ve	
Test +ve	11	5	16
Test -ve	31	58	89
	42	63	105

Sensitivity	$\frac{11}{42}$	26%
Specificity	$\frac{58}{63}$	92%
Accuracy	$\frac{69}{105}$	66%

sensitivity only 26 per cent. How might the sensitivity be increased? Clearly detecting more spleens involved with Hodgkin's disease would increase the examination's sensitivity. If two-thirds of the diseased spleens had been detected, the sensitivity would have been 71 per cent. Nodular disease involving the spleen could not be detected and splenic size was not measured as a volume routinely because of the absence of correlation between size and involvement by Hodgkin's disease if the spleen weighs less than 400 g (Glatstein et al, 1969).

If the accuracy of CT in detecting disease in different abdominal sites other than the spleen is reviewed (Table 8.3) it will be noted that for the liver and para-aortic regions, the next two most common sites of involvement after the spleen, the CT false-positive rate is at least 50 per cent of the true positive rate, 3/5 and 2/4 respectively. Whilst no formal weighting or ranking was employed while assessing the CT examinations both these regions have well established CT criteria for interpretation and therefore it would appear that to relax these further to increase the detection rate would be to increase the false-positive rate to an unacceptable level. The coeliac node regions, the fourth most common site of involvement at laparotomy, had no false-positives because strict criteria were employed in the knowledge that involved nodes are rarely enlarged. Only one significantly enlarged coeliac node was missed by CT but in consequence the false negative rate was high.

Thus it would appear that the relative inability of CT to detect disease in the spleen, liver and unenlarged lymph nodes reflects the limitation of using the criterion of enlargement alone. In this study sensitivity might have been increased but only at the expense of increasing the number of false-positive examinations and thus reducing the specificity to an unacceptable level.

The reliance on morphological criteria for interpretation of the scan pictures emphasises the lack of tissue specificity inherent in the CT technique used in this study. How might tissue specificity be improved?

a. Improved density discrimination: the latest generation scanners may allow better differentiation of normal and abnormal tissue because of improved performance and faster scan times which reduce movement artefact.

b. Use of contrast agents. Conventional intravenous contrast might improve the

64

detection of nodular disease involving the liver and spleen but has limiting problems related to the total dose of contrast and the time required to examine these organs.

The experimental use of an emulsion of iodinated poppyseed oil which is taken up by the Reticulo-endothelial system opacifying the hepatic and splenic parenchyma has been described (Alfidi et al, 1976) but the routine use of organ specific contrast agents is not foreseen in the near future.

c. The use of statistical analysis of CT numbers to characterise tissue: this method has been described to separate normal and cirrhotic levers (Ritchings et al, 1979), but the technique requires areas of tissue 3 cm square and therefore could not be employed with unenlarged lymph nodes.

If one accepts the limitations of CT examination of the abdomen as defined by this study, how may CT be used in the management of lymphomas?

Computed tomography cannot be used as the only abdominal investigation of Hodgkin's disease because of the large numbers of false-negative results in detecting splenic involvement (Table 8.2). Radiotherapy is the treatment of choice for Stages I and II in most centres. As the effectiveness of this treatment depends on knowing that infra-diaphragmatic disease is not present and CT would not detect Stage III disease involving the spleen in most patients, CT may not replace laparotomy unless splenic and total node irradiation and chemotherapy in Stages I and II disease is contemplated.

If CT is compared with lymphography it is seen to be as effective as lymphography in detecting para-aortic lymph node disease (Table 8.4) and has the advantage of detecting disease outside the lymphographic area (Table 8.5). Computed tomography may therefore replace lymphography (Best et al, 1978; Blackledge et al, 1980; Earl et al, 1980). In the Manchester Lymphoma Group Studies of H.D., CT is used routinely as part of the Staging investigation (Fig. 8.1).

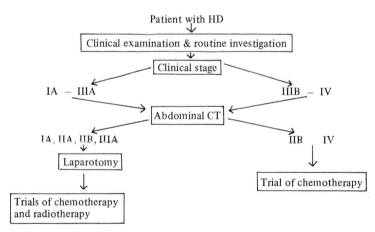

Fig. 8.1 Role of CT in staging and management of patient with Hodgkin's disease.

In the staging of Hodgkin's disease a non-invasive investigation has two potential functions. One is to advance the stage of disease so that invasive techniques such as laparotomy are unnecessary. The other is to establish the extent of disease so that adequate radiation ports can be applied if radiotherapy is the appropriate treatment. In both these respects CT is shown in this study to be superior to lymphography.

Bayes theorem may be applied to different rates of prevalence of H.D. using the sensitivity and specificity for CT examination derived in this study (Table 8.6). The differences between the curves for normal and abnormal tests (Fig. 8.2) is a measure of the information content of the test. It will be seen that the greatest difference for post-test probability is for a prevalence of 0.4, that is 40 per cent, and that the ability to discriminate between disease and no disease is greatest for

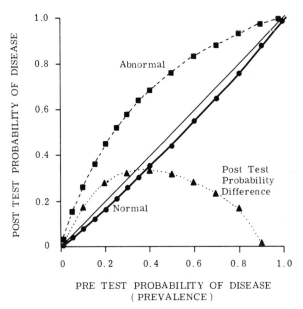

Fig. 8.2 The pre- and post-test probabilities of disease calculated by Bayes theorem are plotted for abnormal and normal CT examination results (specificity 92 per cent, sensitivity 26 per cent). The line with squares defines the relationship for an abnormal test, the line marked with circles defines a normal test. The line marked with triangles marks the difference between both results at different probabilities or prevalence of disease.

prevalence rates below 50 per cent (0.5). It is worth noting that the prevalence of abdominal disease in the selected group of 105 patients who had laparotomy in this study is 40 per cent (42/105). High specificity and low sensitivity are the characteristics of a good screening test for a disease of low prevalence and suggest that CT may be used in this role.

The effect diagnostic examinations have on the financial costs of diagnosis and treatment is complex. Financial costs associated with diagnostic tests must include not only the costs of the tests but also the differences in costs for patients incorrectly treated as a consequence of false negative and false positive results. This discussion may be widened to include, not only the financial consequences but the total consequences for the patient, of errors in testing. Metz (1976) has derived an expression that relates the results of tests and disease prevalence to the average net cost associated with the use of a particular diagnostic test:

$$\bar{C} = \left[C_o + C_{FN}P(D+) + C_{TN}P(D-) \right]$$
$$- \left[C_{FN} - C_{TP} \right] P(T + | D+)P(D+)$$
$$+ \left[C_{FP} - C_{TN} \right] P(T + | D-) P(D-)$$

Where $\bar{C}$ = the average cost of the diagnostic text and the costs of its consequences; C_o = the cost of the test; C_{TP}, C_{FN}, C_{FP}, C_{TN} = the financial costs of the consequences of true positive, false negative, false positive and true negative tests; $P(D+)$ = the disease prevalence; $P(T+| D+)$ = the probability of an abnormal test in the presence of disease and $P(T+| D-)$ = the probability of an abnormal test in the absence of disease.

Inspection of this expression reveals an important point. Whatever the costs of the consequences of the diagnostic test, the average cost $(\bar{C})$ is related to the cost of the test (C_o). Thus, a new test which may produce better decisions and thus reduce the decision consequence costs may, if very expensive, increase the average cost $(\bar{C})$. There therefore may be a real bar to the introduction of a new high cost diagnostic test even with regard to the cost consequences of the decisions it may make.

Metz (1976) has related this expression to ROC analysis, the terms $P(T+| D+)$ and $P(T+ | D-)$ are the same as the True positive fraction (TPF) and the False positive fraction (FPF) which are the co-ordinates of an ROC curve and has derived a further expression:

$$\begin{array}{c} \text{Optimum decision} \\ \text{threshold defined as} \\ \text{the slope at a point} \\ \text{on an ROC curve} \end{array} = \frac{P(D-)}{P(D+)} \quad \times \quad \frac{[C_{FP} - C_{TN}]}{[C_{FN} - C_{TP}]}$$

One may summarise the outcome of this expression simplistically in the following way, the larger the number on the right-hand side of the expression the stricter the criteria that should be used for the interpretation of the test. If one considers the use of a diagnostic test in a disease with a low prevalence where $P(D+)$ is small and $P(D-) = 1-P(D+)$ is large, this will tend to produce a large number on the right and thus require strict criteria. Similarly, if one examines the consequence costs element of the expression, it is noted that if the difference between the costs of a false positive and a true negative decision, $C_{FP} - C_{TN}$ is much greater than the difference between the costs of a false negative and a true positive position $C_{FN} - C_{TP}$ (the situation if further diagnostic tests were harmful and unnecessary, or if treatment could do harm but carried no benefit) the number tends to be large, and thus again strict criteria in the interpretation of the test should be employed. If conversely $C_{FP} - C_{TN}$ is much less than $C_{FN} - C_{TP}$ (as would be the case if further investigation or treatment were harmless but extremely beneficial if required) this reduces the number on the right-hand side suggesting laxer criteria might be employed.

What are the implications of this analysis for the interpretation of CT examinations in patients with Hodgkin's disease? Firstly, it supports the conclusion that CT may be employed as a screening test with the decision threshold currently applied. The incidence of lymphoma is approximately 1 in 20,000 and thus the term P(D–) will be so large as to influence the right-hand side of the expression irrespective of the consequence costs. Secondly, with the prevalence of abdominal disease in the selected group of patients in this study, the prevalence term of the expression is approximately 1 $(\frac{1}{0.4} - 0.4)$ and thus the consequence costs will influence the choice of the decision criteria. If one examines the Stage changes in the 176 patients in this study (Table 8.7) it is noted that no patient has a reduction

Table 8.7 Staging in patients with previously untreated Hodgkin's disease

Clinical stage	Pathological stage						Change of stage as % of total
	1	2	3	4	No/Total %		
1A	43	1	12	3	16/60	27	9
1B	2		1		1/3	33	0.6
2A		32	17	2	19/51	37	11
2B		7	4	4	8/15	53	4.5
3A		1	6		1/7	14	0.6
3B			5		5		
4A				11	11		
4B				25	25		
Total	45	41	45	45	176		

of Stage and there are a total of 45 increases in Stage. In the contest of this study this means, in the majority of changes, the detection of disease in the upper abdomen and this frequently in the spleen. Again, within the context of the study an increase to Stage III will mean that the changes in therapeutic management of the patient are further treatment. This would suggest that laxer criteria should be employed in the interpretation of the CT examination. As previously discussed, however, the criteria already employed cannot be relaxed further because in those areas in the abdomen where there are more diagnostic criteria and therefore the possibility of relaxing the diagnostic threshold there are already large numbers of false positive results. This reinforces the conclusion that to improve the perform-ance of the CT examination, disease in the spleen has to be recognised.

Conclusions

1. CT may replace lymphography as a non-invasive Staging investigation.

2. CT may be used as a screening test for enlarged abdominal lymph nodes.

3. If CT is to be made more sensitive, disease involving the spleen must be detected.

References

Alfidi R J, Lavel-Jeantet M A 1976 A promising contrast agent for computed tomography of the liver and spleen. Radiology 121: 491

68

Best J J, Isherwood I 1977 The Manchester experience. In: Berlin Computerised axial tomography in clinical practice. Springer-Verlag, Berlin p 411

Best J J K, Blackledge G, Forbes W St C, Todd I D H, Eddleston B, Crowther D, Isherwood I 1978 Computed tomography of the abdomen in the staging and clinical management of lymphoma. British Medical Journal 2: 1675–1677

Blackledge G, Best J J K 1980 Computed tomography (CT) in the staging of patients with Hodgkin's Disease: A report on 136 patients. Clinical Radiology 31: 143–147

Carbone P P, Kaplan H S, Musshoff K, Smithers D W, Tubiana M 1971 Report of the committee of Hodgkin's disease classification. Cancer Research 31: 1860–1861

Crowther D, Blackledge G, Best J J K 1979 The role of computed tomography of the abdomen in the diagnosis of staging of patients with lymphoma. Clinics in Haematology 8(3): 567–591

Earl E M, Sutcliffe I, Kelsey-Fry I, Tucker A K, Young J, Husband J, Wrigley P F M, Malpas J S 1980 Computerised tomographic (CT) abdominal scanning in Hodgkin's disease. Clinical Radiology 31: 149–153

Glatstein E, Ward Trueblood H, Enright L P, Rosenberg S A, Kaplan H S, 1970 Surgical staging of abdominal involvement in unselected patients with Hodgkin's disease. Radiology 97: 425–432

Isherwood I, Pullan B R, Ritchings R T 1978 Radiation dose in neuroradiological procedures. Neuroradiology 16: 477–481

Karawada Y, Goldberg L, Brady L, Paulides C, Matsumoto T 1976 Staging laparotomy for Hodgkin's disease. The American Surgeon 42: 332–345

Metz C E, Starr S J, Lusted L B 1976 Quantitative evaluation of visual defection performance in medicine: ROC analysis and determination of diagnostic benefit. In: Hay G A (ed) Medical images: Formation, perception and measurement. Wiley, New York, p 220–241

Ritchings R T, Pullan B R, Lucas S B, Fawcitt R A, Best J J K, Isherwood I, Morris A I 1979 An analysis of the spatial distribution of attenuation valves in computed tomographic scans of liver and spleen. Journal of Computer Assisted Tomography 3(1): 36–39

9. The delineation of head and neck tumours by computed tomography

COLIN PARSONS

The speciality of head and neck oncology is concerned with all tumours arising within that anatomical region excluding the central nervous system. The diagnostic problems which occur are legion particularly now that computed tomography provides structural information, especially of soft tissues, which was not available from other radiological methods. If a diagnostic radiologist is to make any contribution in this field he must thoroughly understand the anatomy so that normal structures are not mistaken for pathology. The tumours with which we are concerned arise in the para-nasal sinuses, naso-pharynx, oro-pharynx, parotid, larynx, the soft tissues and the skull base. This provides a tremendous variety of anatomical situations and variety of tumour morphology, behaviour and response to treatment. The indications for carrying out the CT scan and the precise details of the technique used change accordingly.

The clarity with which abnormalities can be demonstrated is governed by the specification of the CT scanner used. In ideal circumstances, a high resolution format is used for demonstrating the skull base, a short scan time to eliminate movement artefact when examining the larynx and a tilting gantry to facilitate coronal views of the face.

Para-nasal sinuses

Malignant tumours of the para-nasal sinuses account for less than 1 per cent of all cancer and yet comprise a particularly distressing and challenging group of diseases. Less than 10 per cent of patients have local lymph node metastases at presentation and even fewer subsequently exhibit distant spread. It is the local extent of tumour which must be defined accurately so that operability can be determined or the adequacy of radiotherapy fields assessed. Since clinical examination is hampered by the surrounding bony structures, diagnostic radiology has an important part to play. Conventional techniques can demonstrate tumour within the air filled para-nasal sinuses and nasal airways and can show gross bone destruction, but soft tissue tumour extending posteriorly and superiorly from the sinuses is frequently missed. The sites of involvement which are of greatest importance in determining operability are the pterygoid region, naso-pharynx, sphenoid sinus, posterior ethmoid air cells, cribriform plate, orbital apex, and the skull base. Since tumours confined within the sinus produce symptoms identical to benign disease, these important areas are commonly involved by the time the patient is referred to a specialist unit for assessment.

70

Computed tomography offers two major advantages over conventional methods. First, the tomographic technique avoids degradation of the image by overlying structures. Second, CT provides the ability to distinguish between soft tissues of similar density. This enables soft tissue planes in the pterygoid and infratemporal region to be identified (Hesselink et al, 1978). Examination of the sinuses should commence with transverse slices parallel to the anthropomorphic base line starting at the level of the hard palate and proceeding upwards to include the frontal sinuses. 1.3 cm collimation is satisfactory and slices should be obtained at 1 cm intervals. The patient is then turned prone with the chin hyper-extended and coronal sections obtained from the sphenoid sinuses forward to clear the anterior ethmoid air cells. Injection of intravenous contrast medium is usually unhelpful, except for demonstrating intracranial tumour extension (vide infra).

A wide range of histological tumours occur in the paranasal sinuses and, not surprisingly, the aggressiveness of the tumour is reflected in the radiological appearance (Figs 9.1 and 9.2). Sinus opacification is seen in virtually all untreated

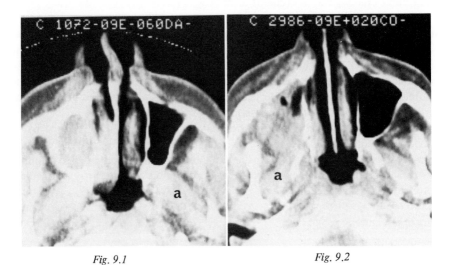

Fig. 9.1   Fig. 9.2

Fig. 9.1 Transverse section through the maxillary antra showing a lymphoma causing sinus opacification and displacement of the bony wall. On the normal side fat planes can be recognised immediately posterior to the antrum and on the anterior surface of the lateral pterygoid muscle (a)

Fig. 9.2 Transverse section through a very aggressive squamous carcinoma of the maxillary antrum which has destroyed the posterior bony wall and extends through the buccal fat plane to invade the anterior surface of lateral pterygoid muscle (a)

patients (Forbes et al, 1978; Parsons & Hodson, 1979; Hesselink, New, Davis et al, 1978). The soft tissue density of the tumour is identical to that of benign mucosal swelling and overlaps with the density of fluid, so that features in addition to opacification are necessary to diagnose malignancy. Opacification of contiguous sinuses may indicate that tumour has spread from one to the other or that an ostium is blocked by the tumour mass, causing the retention of secretions within the other sinus. This is particularly common when tumour extends into the apex of the nasal airway, obstructing the ethmoid air cells. Repeat scans after radiotherapy may give more accurate assessment of tumour extent, the tumour tissue is frequently smaller allowing the ostia to become reopened and re-establishing drainage. In this way, previously opaque sinuses may become re-aerated, so that more accurate assessment of tumour extent is possible.

Tumour extending through the posterior wall of the maxillary antrum can be recognised as a soft tissue density replacing the buccal fat pad, which lies between the antrum and the anterior surface of the lateral pterygoid muscle. Invasion of the pterygoid muscles or temporalis tendon indicates that the tumour is unresectable and its demonstration may save the patient an exploratory operation (Fig. 9.2). Similarly, extension of tumour into the orbit is recognised by replacement of the low density retro-orbital fat by the soft tissue density of tumour. This occurs commonly through the very thin lateral wall of the ethmoid air cells, the lamina papyracea (Fig. 9.3).

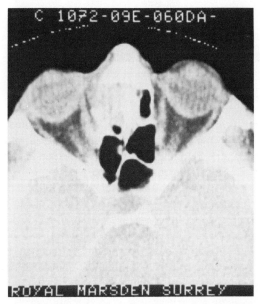

Fig. 9.3 Transverse section through a lymphoma occupying the right anterior ethmoid air cells and extending through the lamina papyracea into the orbit but extending no further than the medial rectus muscle.

The demonstration of tumour extending into the orbit anteriorly but no further than the medial rectus muscle may not preclude ethmoidectomy but permits the surgeon to plan exenteration of the orbit as part of a curative operation. When the orbital apex is involved, however, curative resection is impossible. Whilst replacement of the orbital fat by soft tissue tumour is the earliest sign of involvement, later, displacement of the globe and muscle cone may occur (Fig. 9.4). The addition of coronal views is essential to assess the extension of maxillary antral

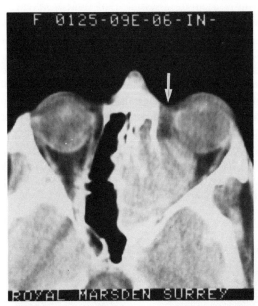

Fig. 9.4 Transverse section through a carcinoma of the ethmoid sinus showing gross orbital involvement displacing the globe laterally. The greater width of retro-orbital fat medial to the globe is apparent (white arrow)

tumours through the orbital floor. A number of bone abnormalities occur. The most common is bone erosion in some parts of the sinus wall, pterygoid plates or skull base (Figs. 9.2 and 9.5). Longstanding slowly expanding tumours displace the sinus wall (Fig. 9.1) and if large enough the nasal septum. Pressure by such longstanding tumours may be associated with clearly defined bone destruction. Sclerosis and thickening of the sinus wall and pterygoid plates may occur when the tumour is associated with infection but has also been seen in two patients with lymphomas but no superadded infection, and after neutron therapy which has destroyed the antrum. New bone formation is found in both benign and malignant primary bone tumours arising within the sinuses. The benign tumours usually show homogenous bone formation and the malignant tumours are usually spicular, have patchy bone deposition, but may also show areas of more uniform bone formation. Although the bony components of such tumours may be very sharply defined there is often an associated diffuse soft tissue mass.

Intravenous contrast injection may cause slight enhancement of paranasal sinus tumours, but this is usually no greater than the enhancement of surrounding muscles, and does not permit further detection of spread within the facial region. However, undiagnosed intracranial extension may be recognised solely as the result of enhancement (Fig. 9.6). Thus, whenever there are physical signs or symptoms suggesting cranial nerve involvement the examination should be extended to at least the lower part of the brain following the injection of intravenous contrast medium.

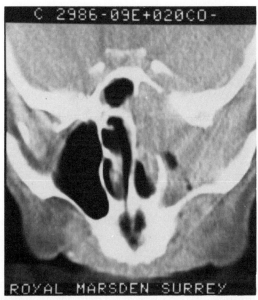

Fig. 9.5 Coronal section through an advanced antral carcinoma extending into the nasal cavity, left half of the sphenoid sinus with destruction of the middle fossa floor.

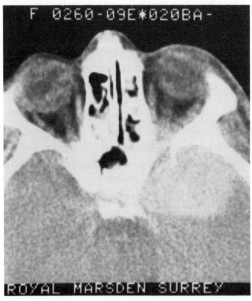

Fig. 9.6 Extension of a very advanced squamous carcinoma through the skull base is revealed by widening of the optic canal and enhancement of intracranial tumour after contrast injection.

The additional information obtained from CT compared with clinical examination and conventional radiology is recorded in Table 9.1. In the paranasal sinus

Table 9.1 Additional information from CT in 32 patients with paranasal sinus tumours

CT findings	No of patients
Extension into pterygoid region	11
Orbital involvement	3
Sphenoid sinus involvement	1

tumours CT provides information which has an important bearing on operability and provides information regarding the extent of resection which is required to effect cure.

The pharynx

Physicians who are not personally concerned with assessing pharyngeal tumours may feel that clinical examination making use of inspection, either directly or with a mirror, and palpation under anaesthesia would provide an accurate assessment of tumour extent. With the demonstration of skull base erosion by conventional radiology there would seem little place for computed tomography to provide additional useful information. However, these methods are notoriously inaccurate for recognising the sub-mucosal limits of tumour and the degree of spread laterally into the para-pharyngeal space. It is often difficult for the examining physician to realise that one wall of the naso-pharynx is uniformly displaced inward. Three very prominent structures are found on the lateral wall of the naso-pharynx, the *Eustachian orifice,* separated from the fossa of *Rosenmuller* by the *salpingopharyngeal fold.* These are encompassed laterally by the superior constrictor which forms the medial boundary of the very important para-pharyngeal space. This extends from the skull base down to the level of the hyoid bone. Once pharyngeal tumour has invaded this fat filled space, spread in a longitudinal direction occurs readily.

On the lateral wall of the oro-pharynx the pillar of the fauces with the intervening tonsil are not as prominent as the recesses and tubal elevation seen in the naso-pharynx. This wall terminates anteriorly in the glosso-tonsillar recess, and is continuous with the lateral pharyngo-epiglottic fold and base of tongue. All these structures are commonly involved by extending tumour. The lateral relation remains the para-pharyngeal space with the same implications for tumour extension as for the naso-pharynx.

CT examination of the nasopharynx should commence with transverse slices from the level of the skull base downward to clear the tumour. Thus, sections as far caudally as the hyoid bone may be required if the para-pharyngeal space is invaded. Once the transverse slices have been satisfactorily completed coronal views are necessary to show small volumes of soft tissue tumour on the roof of the nasopharynx or on the superior surface of the soft palate, and are tremendously useful in assessing skull base erosion. Lymph node involvement by nasopharyngeal tumour is common, occurring in up to 70 per cent of patients at presentation. If there is difficulty in differentiating enlarged lymph nodes from vessels seen in cross-section, then some slices should be repeated after intravenous contrast medium has been given.

On the whole tumours in the naso- and oro-pharynx are usually recognised as a soft tissue mass. False positive interpretation can occur when there is pooling of saliva in the fossa of Rosenmuller or the patient is able to hold the pharynx in an asymmetrical shape. This can be overcome by allowing the patient to swallow and then repeating that tomographic slice. Frequently tumours of this region are advanced at presentation so that the soft tissue mass extends into the para-pharyngeal fat space and may invade the pterygoid muscles and skull base (Fig. 9.7). There is often an excellent response following radiotherapy so that CT may demonstrate a very small volume of residual abnormal soft tissue and the

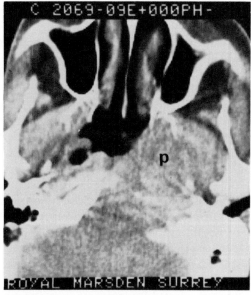

Fig. 9.7 Transverse section through the nasopharynx shows a very advanced tumour occupying the right lateral and posterior walls with gross tumour extension into the parapharyngeal space (P) and bone destruction in the occiput.

radiologist is unable to say whether this contains viable tumour or not, so that, although we can demonstrate an abnormality the significance may not be clear in a single examination and in that case there is a need for serial follow up scans.

Comparison of T staging (Ho, 1978) of nasopharyngeal tumours by conventional techniques and CT would seem to show no great information gain by the newer technique (Table 9.2). However, the quality of the diagnostic information produced is considerably better by CT particularly in the demonstration of parapharyngeal space involvement and the investigation of elderly infirm patients who are unable to maintain the position required for conventional SMV Tomography. In this group of patients (Table 9.2) conventional radiography was however superior at demonstrating minor degrees of bone erosion.

Table 9.2 Nasopharyngeal tumours. Comparison of T-staging

Stage	Conventional methods (No. of patients)	CT (No. of patients)	Stage change Post-CT (No. of patients)
T3	10	10	0
T2	6	7	1
T1	2	1	1
To	5	5	0

The parotid gland

The traditional method of examining the parotid gland includes bimanual palpation, which gives an accurate assessment of the superficial lobe of the gland and will detect gross tumour extension into the pharynx, and sialography, which adds useful information by showing duct displacement by tumour but fails to show the extent of tumour away from the gland itself. Conventional films may show skull base destruction associated with the larger tumours. CT can provide all of this information at one examination and demonstrate the soft tissue extent of tumour more accurately.

CT examination of the parotid should commence below the angle of the mandible and proceed upward to the zygomatic arch, but, these limits may need to be extended to encompass the larger tumours. Intravenous contrast injection may be helpful since many parotid tumours enhance and is also useful for showing the relationship of the tumour to the major vessels prior to surgery.

The parotid gland may be identified as a low density structure (-5 to -15 EMI units) lying immediately posterior and superficial to the masseter muscle and mandible. The deep lobe is triangular in shape with its apex passing medially and forward towards the para-pharyngeal space. The deep posterior relations are the great vessels, the styloid process and its attached muscles, the posterior belly of digastric and the sterno-mastoid muscles. The gland appears very well defined because it is enclosed in a fascial sheath; this is attached above to the zygomatic arch and below separates the parotid from the submandibular salivary gland.

All the parotid tumours referred for investigation in our department have been huge, disrupting the fascial sheath and filling the parapharyngeal space and the pterygoid region. The route of forward extension of deep parotid tumours is determined by the bone of the mandible lying laterally and the maxilla medially, so that tumour extends forward to the cheek between these bony limits. Destruction of the pterygoid plates and posterior wall of the maxillary antrum may occur or the tumour may spread upward through the para-pharyngeal space to erode the skull base. The contrast provided by fat planes within the face defines the limits of tumour but this may be even more clearly shown following intravenous contrast medium. The larger parotid tumours encircle the great vessels.

Although tumours of the sub-mandibular salivary glands are extremely rare it is important to recognise the normal anatomy of these structures so that it is not confused with pathology. The normal glands are well defined ovoid soft tissue structures immediately lateral to the tongue at the level of the hyoid bone. There is considerable enhancement after injection of intravenous contrast making differentiation from lymph nodes simple. Care must be taken however when examining oro-pharyngeal tumours not to confuse the enhancement in the sub-mandibular salivary glands for extension of oro-pharyngeal tumour into the tongue.

The larynx

CT investigation of laryngeal tumours has been relatively neglected. This is partly due to the ease of physical examination supported by conventional radiology, and, to the fact that some subtle increase in tumour volume demonstrated by CT is unlikely to change radiotherapy treatment fields. It is also partly due to movement artefact when a 20 second scan time is used and to the summation of structures within a 1.3 cm slice width. However, there is a real place for CT in pre-operative assessment.

The larynx is examined with the patient supine and the neck extended during quiet breathing so that the cords are retracted. The cords will not abduct, of course, after a tracheostomy. An infusion of contrast medium during the procedure will cause an increase in density of the thyroid gland enabling its invasion or displacement by laryngeal tumour to be recognised even when the thyroid cartilage is poorly ossified. The contrast medium also shows the relationship of vascular structures to the tumour and facilitates differentiation from lymph nodes seen in cross section. Tomographic slices are obtained at 0.5 cm intervals from the cricoid cartilage to the hyoid bone.

A good deal of anatomical information is available by computed tomography which cannot be obtained by conventional methods (Mancuso et al, 1978), the most important of these is the demonstration of fibro-fatty tissue in the pre-epiglottic space which lies between the hyoid bone and the anterior surface of the epiglottis. The transverse plane allows comparison between the right and left halves of the larynx so that a difference in width of the epiglottis, ary-epiglottic fold or transverse diameter of the various cords can be recognised. Similarly, displacement of the arytenoid cartilages is clearly displayed. The ala of the thyroid cartilage is shown to comprise two cortical layers enabling a minor degree of erosion of the inner surface to be recognised. Similarly, the whole signet of the cricoid cartilage can be identified, presence of invasion of this structure by tumour is vital information before conservative laryngectomy.

In the epiglottis, tumour causes thickening, surface irregularity, with soft tissue extension into the pre-epiglottic fat (Fig. 9.8). Detection of extension into the ary-epiglottic folds is simplified by the transverse plane allowing comparison of one side with the other. The most extensive laryngeal tumours are commonly associated with gross oedema, so that it may prove impossible to be sure where tumour ends and oedema begins. Smooth bilateral symmetrical swelling is usually due to oedema. CT does provide a clear indication of the area of the remaining airway and allows examination of the larynx at a lower level when in these circumstances clinical examination is impossible.

The diagnostic criteria for the diagnosis of tumour involvement of the false or true cords by CT are either enlargement of the cord or irregularity of its medial

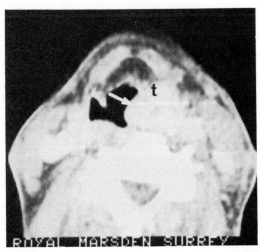

Fig. 9.8 Transverse section through the epiglottis immediately below the level of the hyoid bone shows a large tumour mass occupying the right pyriform sinus extending forward into the pre-epiglottic fat.

border. Only an absolutely sharp medial border of a vocal cord should be accepted as normal (Fig. 9.9). Small volume tumours occupying the superior or inferior

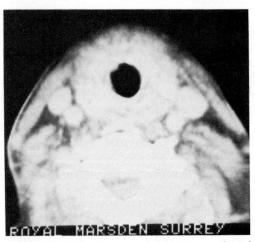

Fig. 9.9 Transverse section through a tumour of right true vocal cord. Only an absolutely sharp medial margin of the vocal cord can be accepted as normal. Quite a small volume of tumour is readily apparent when it occurs on the medial margin but would be missed on the superior or inferior surface of a cord in the transverse plane of CT.

surface of a cord will go undetected, so that minor degrees of subglottic extension have proved very difficult to demonstrate in the transverse plane, due to averaging of density throughout the 1.3 cm of the slice width. For the same reason invasion of the ventricle has had to be assumed whenever tumour involved both the adjacent cords. The acute angle at which the cords meet at the anterior commissure can only be demonstrated in the transverse plane.

Spread of even small volumes of tumour across the midline can be shown by CT at either the anterior or posterior commissures. This is a considerable advantage of the technique and is of value when considering the possibility of vertical hemi-laryngectomy. The extent of invasion across the midline is important when deciding the feasibility of such a procedure. Uniform prominence of a vocal cord may be due to tumour, oedema or paresis with no radiological features to differentiate one from the other, although tumour most commonly produces surface irregularity. Prominence of a vocal cord may also be caused by inward collapse of the thyroid cartilage due to radio-necrosis.

CT provides information which is complementary to conventional radiology and clinical assessment but CT is superior to both of these modalities for showing deep tumour infiltration, cartilage invasion and extension into the soft tissues (Mancuso & Hanafee, 1978) (Fig. 9.10). The information obtained is of great

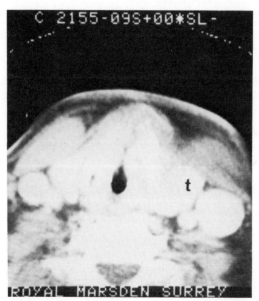

Fig. 9.10 Transverse section through a tumour occupying the anterior two-thirds of each true vocal cord causing perforation of the thyroid cartilage anteriorly. The right upper pole of the thyroid gland (t) is displaced laterally by tumour.

importance in planning conservative laryngectomy (Parsons et al, 1980), the features shown by CT which are important in this respect are shown in Table 9.3.

In the head and neck CT does provide diagnostic information which is not available from clinical examination nor from conventional radiology. This information is easily acquired and has an important bearing on treatment selection.

80

Table 9.3 Features at CT which may influence the surgical procedure

---

1. Pre-epiglottic space involvement
2. Cartilage involvement:
   a. thyroid cartilage invasion or perforation
   b. hyoid bone encirclement
   c. arytenoid displacement
   d. cricoid invasion
3. Extension across anterior or posterior commissure
4. Invasion of adjacent structures:
   a. hypopharynx
   b. thyroid gland
5. Sub-glottic extension

References

Forbes W St C, Fawcitt R A, Isherwood I, Webb R, Farrington T 1978 Computed tomography in the diagnosis of diseases of the paranasal sinuses. Clinical Radiology 29: 501–511

Hesselink J R, New P F J, Davis K R, Weber A L, Robertson G H, Traveras J M 1978 Computed tomography of the paranasal sinuses and face: Part 1. Normal anatomy. Journal of Computer Assisted Tomography 2: 559–567

Hesselink J R, New P F J, Davis K R, Weber A L, Robertson G H, Traveras J M 1978 Computed tomography of the paranasal sinuses and face: Part 2. Pathological anatomy. Journal of Computer Assisted Tomography 2: 568–576

Mancuso A A, Calcaterra T C, Hanafee W N 1978 Computed tomography of the larynx. Radiological Clinics of North America XVI: 195–208

Mancuso A A, Hanafee W N 1978 A comparative evaluation of computed tomography and laryngography; Radiology 133: 131–138

Parsons C, Hodson N 1979 Computed tomography of paranasal sinus tumours. Radiology 132: 641–645

Parsons C, Chapman P, Counter R T, Grundy A 1980 The role of computed tomography in tumours of the larynx. Clinical Radiology (in press)

10. The clinical value of CT in the staging and localisation of pelvic tumours

NEIL HODSON, JANET HUSBAND and PAULINE HOBDAY

Introduction

Optimal radiation therapy can only be delivered if accurate information is available regarding tumour size, location and relationship of the mass to adjacent normal structures. However, full clinical assessment and conventional imaging techniques frequently fail to provide adequate information and this may lead to errors in radiotherapy planning and subsequent treatment failure. To avoid such errors treatment volumes are often made unnecessarily large. Although this policy ensures that the tumour is encompassed within the selected high dose zone, there is an associated rise in attendant morbidity or failure to attain a tumour sterilizing dose.

Computed tomography (CT) now provides the radiotherapist with an imaging technique which will give information about the extent of tumour spread and can also be used directly for radiotherapy planning. The advantages of CT are therefore enormous, but it is essential that its value in clinical practice is assessed critically by comparing the diagnostic information obtained and tumour localisation data with conventional methods which have hitherto been the only techniques available. For this reason, a two part study was designed to evaluate the ability of CT to provide additional diagnostic information in staging of patients with pelvic malignancy and to assess the value of the CT data in radiotherapy treatment planning. In this paper the results of these studies is described and the impact of CT in the radiotherapy management of pelvic malignancy is discussed.

Patients and methods

Between August 1977 and January 1980 over 500 patients with primary pelvic tumours have been investigated using an EMI General Purpose Scanner (CT 5005). A total of 635 CT examinations were carried out. Table 10.1 shows the number of patients scanned in various groups according to tumour type. Most CT examinations were performed in patients with bladder cancer and carcinoma of the cervix. The miscellaneous group consists of patients with primary bone tumours and with soft tissue sarcomas arising in the pelvis. These patients were all scanned in an attempt to obtain further diagnostic information than was already available. High quality images are essential if errors in interpretation are to be avoided and for this reason the patients were all scanned with a full bladder. In addition a water soluble contrast medium was given both orally and rectally before the

Table 10.1 CT – pelvis (August 1977 - January 1980)

Tumour site	No. of patients scanned	Follow-up scans	(%)	Treatment planning scans
Bladder	154	38	(25)	76
Cervix	113	34	(30)	11
Corpus	19	2	(11)	–
Ovary	82	15	(18)	–
Prostate	23	4		18
Rectum	80	32	(40)	15
Miscellaneous	29	10	(34)	9
Total	500	135	(27)	129 (26%)

examination to opacify as much of the bowel as possible. In order to reduce motion artefacts from gas in moving bowel an anticholinergic agent (hyoscine-N-butylbromide 20 mg) was given intramuscularly. Female patients were asked to insert a vaginal tampon to delineate the vaginal vault.

Out of a total of 500 patients, 129 proved suitable for entry into the second part of the study in which CT information was compared with that obtained from conventional methods of treatment planning. Patients were only included in this study if radical radiotherapy was considered appropriate. Patients being planned for large volume regional therapy were not included (e.g. the majority of patients with gynaecological cancer are usually planned with large volumes encompassing the whole pelvis and/or abdomen), because we considered that the potential advantage of precise tumour localisation with CT was unnecessary.

Table 10.1 shows the number of patients in each tumour type entered into the planning study. Radiotherapy plans were produced using all available diagnostic information from clinical examination, conventional radiographs, isotope and ultrasound examinations, and surgical findings. The volume to be treated was localised using a radiotherapy simulator and transferred to a body contour obtained using plaster of Paris strips or malleable wire. CT-integrated therapy planning was carried out independently on the same patients. The techniques employed and the method of CT data transfer directly to the planning computer are described in detail elsewhere (Hobday et al, 1979). Scans were carried out using a flat platter instead of the usual dish-shaped couch. The patient was placed in the therapy position. In patients with bladder cancer slices were repeated through the treatment area with the bladder empty.

Although these images are frequently of poor diagnostic quality they exactly simulate the internal pelvic anatomy during treatment. After the CT examination was completed the scans were reviewed and appropriate CT sections chosen for planning purposes. The CT scan data was transferred by floppy disc to the prototype TP1A Planning System or more recently the EMIPLAN 7000 System. The parameters of tumour localisation, body contour and position of relevant internal structures were then compared with those derived from conventional investigations.

The effect of tissue inhomogeneity corrections in the pelvis were analysed in three different sized patients; small, medium and large stature. Corrected plans were produced using a pixel-by-pixel correction technique (Parker et al, 1979) and the midpoint doses of the bladder and rectum compared with those obtained with no tissue correction. The influence of changing the patient's position from supine to prone and of altering the field arrangement on density correction was also examined. The magnitude of dosimetry changes is influenced by the amount of dense bone and subcutaneous fat within the CT sections. These factors were taken into account by measuring the dose at the level of the femoral neck, 1 cm above the acetabulum and at the level of the first sacral notch.

Results

Diagnostic information

CT findings for each tumour type were compared with the clinical T stage (loco-regional tumour spread), lymphography (N stage, nodal spread) and wherever possible with the surgical specimen (P stage). This comparison with staging was, of course, only possible in those patients examined at presentation. Previously treated patients were evaluated in terms of tumour detection and delineation. According to these parameters an attempt has been made to quantify the additional information provided by CT. The number of patients in whom additional information was provided by CT are shown in Table 10.2. It is beyond the scope

Table 10.2 Diagnostic information gain — Pelvis

Tumour	No. of patients	Major additional information	% patients with gain
Bladder	75	Staging — extravesical spread	57
Cervix	43	Staging — advanced parametrial disease Delineation of recurrence	28
Prostate	19	Staging — gross extracapsular extension	26
Rectum	32	Delineation of tumour recurrence	75
Lymph Nodes	92	Demonstration of unopacified nodes	10

of this text to discuss the detailed results of these comparative studies. Reports of our findings in patients with carcinoma of the bladder and carcinoma of the rectum have already been published (Hodson et al, 1979; Husband et al, 1979).

Briefly, in patients with carcinoma of the *bladder* the major advantage of CT is the ability to demonstrate deep tumour infiltration into the perivesical tissues. (Fig. 10.1). In this group of 75 patients extravesical tumour spread was demonstrated in 3 out of 14 patients who were conventionally stage T2 and 26 out of 36 patients who had been staged as having T3 tumours (UICC Classification, 1978). In the remaining 13 patients the extra information with CT included demonstration of organ involvement or extension of tumour to the pelvic side wall.

84

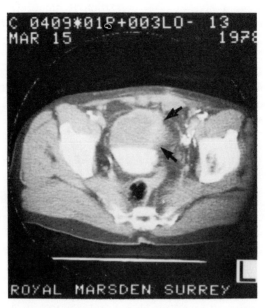

Fig. 10.1 CT scan of a patient with carcinoma of the bladder. The soft tissue tumour on the left bladder wall is seen extending into the perivesical tissues. (arrows).

The information gained in patients with carcinoma of the cervix was, not surprisingly, considerably less than in patients with carcinoma of the bladder. The main reasons are that tumour within the cervix cannot be distinguished from normal surrounding tissue and that the longitudinal axis of the gynaecological organs causes difficulties in interpretation in the cross-sectional plane. Thus, early parametrial spread is difficult or impossible to identify. For example, a large tumour contained within the cervix (Stage IB) cannot be distinguished from an early IIB tumour spreading into the paravesical tissues (FIGO Classification, UICC 1978). Since the attenuation values of the uterus, cervix and vagina are similar spread of tumour upwards into the uterus or downwards into the vagina is not readily appreciated. In more advanced cases, however, CT is more valuable since tumour extension as far as the pelvic wall (Stage IIIB) can be distinguished from earlier degrees of spread (Fig. 10.2). In the comparison of clinical staging with CT staging in 34 new patients with carcinoma of the cervix, additional information was obtained in 7. CT appears to have a more useful role in confirming the presence of recurrent tumour in patients who have been irradiated. In nineteen patients with symptoms suggestive of recurrence, CT demonstrated the mass in 5 and in the remaining 14 patients CT was negative. Twelve of these have remained alive and well for periods of at least one year and two have died of distant metastatic spread. Thus, CT provided further diagnostic information in cervical cancer in 12 out of 43 patients (28 per cent).

In patients with recurrent *rectal* tumours CT provides an excellent method of detecting suspected masses and of delineating the site and size of a known mass.

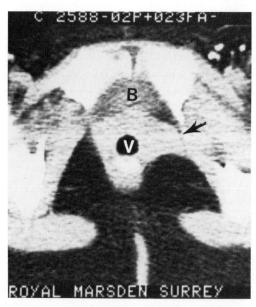

Fig. 10.2 CT scan of a patient with carcinoma of the cervix. Tumour is seen extending from the vagina (V) to the left pelvic wall (arrows). The bladder base is seen anteriorly (B).

Since these masses are difficult to demonstrate by conventional techniques, particularly after abdomino-perineal resection, CT provides additional information in a large proportion of patients. In our series of 32 patients there was diagnostic gain using CT in 75 per cent of cases. A detailed analysis of this series has already been published (Husband et al, 1980).

Assessment of *prostatic* cancer with CT is subject to the same problems as the assessment of cervical cancer; namely, tumour within the gland cannot be distinguished from normal prostatic tissues. Further problems arise because there is a very thin layer of fat between the prostatic capsule and the levator ani muscles making interpretation of tumour infiltration into this space difficult unless disease is advanced. For these reasons we have performed relatively few scans in patients with prostatic cancer; the diagnostic information gain in this group was 4 out of 19 (21 per cent).

Lymph node metastases from pelvic cancers are common. Lymphography is an excellent technique for demonstrating these deposits because they tend to produce little, if any, nodal enlargement and in our opinion lymphography is superior to CT because it demonstrates the internal architecture of the nodes. We have compared the results of CT with lymphography in 92 patients suffering from various types of pelvic cancer. Detailed analysis of these findings is shortly to be published (Husband et al, 1981). In summary, CT is less sensitive than lymphography but may occasionally be useful if lymphography fails for technical reasons, or if the technique is contra-indicated CT is also useful for defining the size and precise site of a mass which has been unopacified by lymphographic contrast medium. In our series, additional useful information was obtained using CT in 10 per cent of patients.

Comparison of CT and conventional tumour localisation

Body contour

Conventional and CT- body contours have been compared in a total group of 129 patients entered into the planning study. The results are shown in Table 10.3. A

Table 10.3 Body contour changes

Alteration in body outline ($\geqslant 1$ cm)		15/129	(12%)
Significant changes	$\geqslant 5\%$ change in MPD or Inadequate tumour coverage	2/129	(1.5%)

discrepancy in body contour was considered significant if equal or greater than 1 cm. Such discrepancy was found in 15 out of 129 (12 per cent) of patients. The effect of these discrepancies on the midpoint tumour dose (MPD) was measured. A change in MPD of more than 5 per cent was noted in one patient and considered clinically important. In another patient an outline error affected the position of the isocentre and led to inadequate tumour coverage.

Tumour localisation

In 23 patients (18 per cent) the proposed conventional target volume did not encompass the tumour adequately as assessed with CT. A larger number of errors occurred using conventional localisation methods in patients with recurrent rectal tumours than in any other site which reflect the increased diagnostic gain obtained with CT. (Fig. 10.3). Table 10.4 shows the number of patients in each tumour

Table 10.4 Adequacy of tumour coverage

Tumour	No. of patients	Coverage inadequate	%
Bladder	76	10	13
Prostate	18	4	22
Rectum	15	4	27
Cervix	11	2	18
Miscellaneous	9	3	
Total	129	23	18

group in which tumour coverage was compared. The number of patients with each tumour in which coverage was found to be inadequate is also shown.

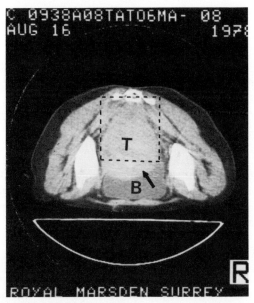

Fig. 10.3 Large recurrent rectal tumour (T). The patient was scanned in the prone position for planning purposes. The tumour extends beyond the proposed treatment volume using conventional methods of localisation (dotted lines).

Tissue inhomogeneities

The maximum percentage change in the midpoint doses of the bladder and rectum for large and small patients are shown in Table 10.5. Maximum percentage change

Table 10.5 Maximum percentage change with CT correction

Position	Technique	Parallel opposed	Four fields	Three fields
Supine	Small	0%	1%	1%
	Large	0%	2%	2%
Prone	Small	0%	0%	-2%
	Large	0%	2%	-4%

Uncorrected minus CT corrected

for all combinations of patient size, field arrangement and cross-sectional level in the supine position was 2 per cent. Table 10.5 also illustrates percentage change recorded at a single point when patients were planned in the prone position. In this situation maximum percentage change for all the combinations studied was 4 per cent. These results are applicable only to the use of 8MeV X-rays but changes of a similar magnitude were recorded for Co^{60} beams.

Treatment volume changes

Table 10.6 shows the changes in treatment volume which resulted from the discrepancies found in tumour coverage. Thus, all 23 patients in whom tumour

Table 10.6 Treatment volume alterations

Increased only	13
Increased and moved	6
Moved only	4
Reduced	2
Total	25

coverage was assessed to be inadequate on the basis of CT had treatment volume changes. In 19 patients the treatment volume was increased and in a further 4 patients the treatment volume was simply moved. In 2 patients the treatment volume was reduced.

Discussion

The results of these studies indicate that CT has already made an important impact in the diagnosis and radiotherapy planning of patients with pelvic malignancy. Clearly the value of the technique as a diagnostic tool varies according to tumour type. For example, in carcinoma of the bladder and recurrent rectal tumours CT is probably the best method yet available for demonstrating the soft tissue extent of tumour. Several other studies also indicate that CT is superior to conventional methods of staging in bladder cancer (Seidelmann et al, 1978; Kellett et al, 1980). However, in our series of patients CT was less helpful in the staging of carcinoma of the cervix and prostate. Our results comparing CT with lymphography in the pelvis are disappointing but in general agree with the findings of Lee et al (1978).

The second part of this study has shown that the information provided by CT has significantly altered radiotherapy treatment planning in 19 per cent of patients, of these 23 changes were due to inadequate tumour coverage (18 per cent). These figures are considerably lower than those reported in other studies. Thus, Munzenrider et al (1977) report that tumour coverage of pelvic tumours was inadequate or marginal in 6 out of 17 (35 per cent) of patients investigated. Goitein et al (1979) also found that CT revealed inadequate tumour coverage in over 30 per cent of their pelvic cases. These differences are perhaps surprising since our study was restricted whenever possible to patients planned with small volume treatment. However, there are many variable factors in a comparative study. These include the different treatment policies adopted in a particular centre, the quality of conventional tumour assessment and the selection of patients included in the study.

It is clear from our study and from those of other investigators that CT information provides the opportunity to execute more accurate radiotherapy planning than has previously been possible. Furthermore, it opens the way to an individualised approach so that plans may be optimised according to the particular clinical problem. The influence of improved radiation planning on local tumour control remains unknown but in our view the increased accuracy of CT-therapy planning is a significant advance in clinical practice.

Acknowledgements

We are most grateful to our clinical colleagues for referring their patients to us. The help of Mrs D. Mears and Mrs J. Sangway in scanning the patients and of Mrs Janice O'Donnell and Mrs Rosemary Sewell in preparing the typescript is greatly appreciated.

References

Goitein M, Wittenberg J, Mendiondo M, Doucette J, Friedberg C, Ferrucci J, Gunderson L, Linggood R, Shipley W U, Fineberg H V 1979 The value of CT scanning in radiation therapy treatment planning: a prospective study. International Journal of Radiation Oncology Biology Physics (in press)

Hobday P, Hodson N J, Husband J E, Parker R P, Macdonald J S 1979 Computed tomography applied to radiotherapy treatment planning: techniques and results. Radiology 133: 477

Hodson N J, Husband J E, Macdonald J S 1979 The role of computed tomography in the staging of bladder cancer. Clinical Radiology 30: 389-395

Husband J E, Hodson N J, Parsons C A 1980 Computed tomography in recurrent rectal tumours. Radiology 134: 677-682

Kellett M J, Kelsey Fry I, Husband J E, Oliver T D 1980 CT scanning as an adjunct to bimanual examination for staging of bladder tumours. British Journal of Urology 52: 101-106

Lee J K T, Stanley R J, Sagel S S, McLennan B L 1978 Accuracy of computed tomography in detecting intra-abdominal and pelvic lymph node metastases from pelvic cancers. American Journal of Roentgenology 131: 675-679

Munzenrider J E, Pilepich M, Rene-Ferrero J B, Tchakarova I, Carter B L 1977 Use of body scanner in radiotherapy treatment planning. Cancer 40(1): 170-179

Parker R P, Hobday P A, Cassell K J 1979 The direct use of CT numbers in radiotherapy dosage calculations for inhomogeneous media. Physics Medicine Biology 24(4): 802-809

Seidelmann F E, Cohen W N, Bryan P J, Temes S P, Kraus D, Schoenrock G 1978 Accuracy of CT staging of bladder neoplasms using the gas-filled method: Report of twenty-one patients with surgical confirmation. American Journal of Roentgenology 130: 735-739

U.I.C.C. (International Union Against Cancer) 1978 TNM classification of malignant tumours, 3rd ed.

11. CT scanning in radiotherapy treatment planning: its strengths and weaknesses

R. P. PARKER and P. A. HOBDAY

Introduction

If the use of expensive equipment such as CT scanners and CT-linked treatment planning computers is to be justified, decisions must be made after consideration of both the strengths and weaknesses of such a system. As an introduction to the section on the application of CT to treatment planning, various questions will therefore be posed and answers suggested. The overall treatment planning process is shown schematically (Fig. 11.1) and the stages where CT can help are indicated.

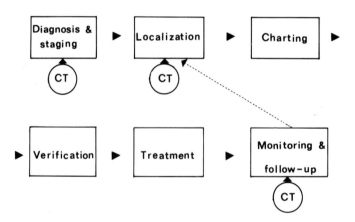

Fig. 11.1 Schematic diagram of treatment planning process.

The process starts with diagnosis and staging: it is only after the tumour extent has been established that the target volume can be mapped out and a suitable arrangement of beams calculated. CT provides excellent images of diagnostic quality. Providing precautions are taken to position the patient in the treatment position (Hobday et al, 1979) throughout the CT examination, then localisation of the target volume can also be obtained on the same occasion.

With the introduction of a new imaging modality such as CT it is likely that the assistance of a radiologist will be required in interpreting the picture and marking out the visible extent of the tumour. The radiotherapist can then establish the target volume and the physicist calculate a suitable isodose distribution. Clearly this is best achieved by a group, and at the Royal Marsden Hospital we are fortunate in being able to operate as an interdisciplinary planning team with expert technical assistance.

When is it useful?

Ideally, this question would be answered by a clinical trial conducted with and without CT. However, this is impracticable. Measurement of tumour response may be a substitute, at least in the short term, and several chapters in this book are devoted to this important topic (see Husband et al, this volume). At the present time we, in common with a number of other centres, have opted to compare the localisation and tumour extent obtained with and without the assistance of CT. The results on our first 50 patients were reported at the end of 1977 (Macdonald et al, 1977) and later extended to 123 patients (Hobday et al, 1979). The series now amounts to 289 patients and the cumulative results are summarised here and referred to as RMH 80. Only those changes regarded as significant are reported, namely those in which there is inadequate tumour coverage due to field size or position or when the mid-point tumour dose is altered by more than 5 per cent. Where possible our results are compared with publications from other groups, although their figures are not always expressed in similar terms. Other papers in this volume also provide up-to-date data for comparison.

Table 11.1 Major plan alterations due to CT

Tufts	1977	45% of 75 patients
Mallinckrodt	1978	20% of 45 patients
Brizel	1979	30% of 72 patients (pelvis)
MGH	1979	36% of 77 patients
RMH	1980	25% of 289 patients

Table 11.1 lists the number of major plan alterations due to CT that we have made, together with those published from Tufts University (Tufts '77) by Munzenrider et al, the Mallinckrodt Radiotherapy Department (Ragan & Perez, 1978), results for the pelvis by Brizel et al (1979) from Hollywood, Florida and a recent series from Massachusetts General Hospital (MGH '79) reported by Goitein et al. Considering the differences in patient selection and technique that are to be expected there is a notable agreement between the various centres.

The alterations in plans may be considered under several categories. CT provides excellent information on the patient outline and in the RMH study this has been compared with that obtained by the usual methods of lead wire or plaster of Paris bandage. The number of significant changes was not in excess of 2 per cent except for the abdomen, where it amounted to 7 per cent. It would therefore appear that conventional outlining techniques are satisfactory.

CT also gives anatomical data on the location of normal, radio-sensitive organs. In the RMH series discrepancies between conventional and CT localisation were notably for the kidneys in the abdomen (29 per cent), and the spinal cord in the thorax (9 per cent). In both instances the changes were primarily ascribed to poor visualisation of these organs on the conventional A-P and lateral X-radiographs.

Better imaging of involved tissue with CT can result in both enlargement and movement of the treatment field, and so avoid inadequate tumour coverage.

Table 11.2 Inadequate tumour coverage

	Tufts '77	MGH '79	RMH '80
Pelvis	6%	32%	16%
Abdomen	36%	34%	57%
Thorax	24%	25%	25%
Head and neck	–	–	18%
Total	15%	35%	21%

Table 11.2 summarises the incidence of such alterations; the main differences between the Radiotherapy Centres can be explained by patient selection. For example, in their 1977 series, Tufts were using large fields in the pelvis, resulting in few instances of inadequate tumour coverage. By contrast, the MGH '79 results include many changes to small, boost fields. The RMH '80 figures for the abdomen are somewhat distorted due to an unusual proportion (47 per cent) of Ca pancreas, a tumour notoriously difficult to image by conventional means.

If large treatment fields have been planned conventionally due to difficulties in precise localisation, then the extra information provided by CT allows a reduction in field size. At our own hospital this only occurred to a significant extent (18 per cent) in the abdomen, compared with an overall total of 24 per cent for Tufts 77 and 11 per cent for MGH 79.

In summary, most changes are due to better visualisation and localisation. In the RMH series these primarily resulted in increased field sizes in the pelvis and head and neck, whilst in the abdomen and thorax there are about equal numbers of increased and moved fields. It must be emphasised that to achieve these results, good diagnostic quality CT scans are required. Images of lower quality, in whatever anatomical plane they are obtained, will not demonstrate the increased tumour extent or subtleties of anatomical structure which are so significant in affecting the treatment plans. Visualisation of the normal anatomy ranks next in importance. Here the strength of CT must be considered in relation to other localising techniques such as ultrasound. In a smaller number of cases field sizes have actually been reduced after CT-assisted planning; with increasing confidence and more use of boost fields, the importance of this last group is likely to grow.

How does it affect dosimetry?

Corrections for the varying attenuation of X-rays by different tissue types may be carried out automatically using algorithms based on the actual values of the CT numbers. Chapters by Cunningham and Dutreix in this volume consider such calculations in detail, and we ourselves have developed methods on our EMIPLAN treatment planning computer which are described elsewhere (Parker et al, 1979 and 1980).

For photons the corrections are most important in the thorax, where differences in mid-point tumour dose between corrected and uncorrected plans lie in the range 10-25 per cent. As well as considering tumour dose it is instructive to examine the overall changes in the dose distribution.

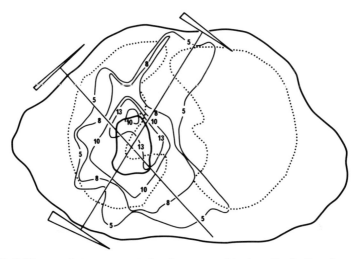

Fig. 11.2 Differences between corrected and uncorrected isodose distributions for a three-field bronchus technique using 8 MeV photons.

Figure 11.2 illustrates the *differences* between the corrected and uncorrected plans for a 3-field bronchus treatment with 8 MeV photons. The decrease in dose homogeneity in the target volume and the increased dose to the spinal cord are noticeable. At present, most of the effort in using CT data to correct isodose distributions for inhomogeneities have been devoted to photon beams. However such corrections are more important for high energy electron beams, where the alteration in electron range can result in changes of 100 per cent to dose estimates. This is beginning to receive attention by a number of groups (for example, Dutreix, this volume) and it is to be hoped that the application of inhomogeneity corrections, together with the use of compensators to adjust the dose distribution, will give radiotherapists more confidence in the application of this modality.

What limits the accuracy?

The overall accuracy in administering radiotherapeutic treatment will be affected by both the equipment and the patient. This has been considered in general terms by ICRU (1976), and in relation to CT-scanning by Parker (1980).

It is necessary to consider inaccuracies both in dose estimates and anatomical location. If inhomogeneity corrections are applied using the CT-data then the inaccuracy in dose estimates for photons is at best in the range $2.5 - 7.5$ per cent, and can be improved by further refinement of the algorithms, particularly near to interfaces.

Using a CT-linked treatment planning system data are transferred digitally. the spatial accuracy is therefore limited in the plane of the slice by the resolution of the scanner, which in turn depends on the contrast of the structure imaged. In

94

the longitudinal direction the resolution is governed by the slice width which may be up to 15 mm, although much narrower slices are now available.

The improved localisation due to CT does, however, relate only to the patient at that particular time, and as set up on the scanner. Whilst normal care is taken to ensure reproducibility of position at scanning, verification and daily treatment, it is appropriate to question the accuracy by which this is achieved (Byhardt et al, 1978). In an attempt to quantify this, a group of skilled radiographers took turns in setting up a series of patients a number of times and recording the distances between skeletal landmarks and a tattoo placed over bone. Any variation will be due to a combination of lack of reproducibility in position and difficulty in defining the landmark.

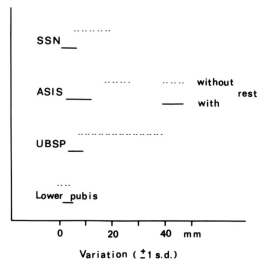

Fig. 11.3 Reproducibility of patient positioning.

Figure 11.3 illustrates the results for sternal notch (SSN), anterior superior iliac spines (ASIS), upper border of symphysis pubis (UBSP) and root of penis or commissure of labia (lower pubis). The horizontal lines represent ± standard deviation for the variations recorded by the radiographers. The study was repeated using a prototype head and arm rest devised by Mr M. Heavens of EMI Medical Ltd. Clearly this improves positioning significantly, but only SSN and lower pubis have mean values less than 5 mm. It is concluded that positioning aids are essential and that provided landmarks are used which are well defined and fixed in relation to the underlying anatomy, a reproducibility of 5 mm is possible. If no aids are used, variations of 10–20 mm are likely.

Using SSN and lower pubis, together with the head and arm rest, one radiographer repeated the same patient a number of times over a period of some weeks. An analysis of the results for various patients indicates that reproducibility better than 5 mm can be obtained. It must be emphasised, however, that these patients were relatively fit. The study relates to external landmarks only and no attention has been paid to possible rotation of the body. These results are to be compared with a precision of $\pm$ 1 mm for a simulator, linear accelerator and a CT scanner in the plane of the slice. In the longitudinal direction scanner accuracy is governed by slice width, couch scales, backlash in couch movements and difficulty in defining the centre of the slice. At the present stage of development, reproducibility of scanner and patient in the longitudinal direction requires improvement.

Which patients will benefit?

Whilst in any individual case the decision to implement CT-based treatment planning must be a clinical one, the strengths and weaknesses of the technique as outlined above enable the selection of certain categories of patients as likely to benefit.

In the various series summarised in Table 11.1, patients were selected on the basis of treatment with radical intent. Clearly a better knowledge of tumour extent, together with good localisation and accurate dose calculations, will improve the treatment. It is, of course, too early to say whether this results in better survival rates.

We know of no reported studies regarding patients undergoing palliative treatments. Many of these are treated with large fields, and more accurate localisation and delineation of the tumour is unlikely to improve the treatment significantly. Good localisation of normal, radiosensitive tissues may be advisable, and our results in the thorax and abdomen suggest that conventional methods are in need of some improvement. More accurate dose calculations will result from the quantitative anatomical data available from a CT scan, but this will primarily affect thorax treatments, and will it result in a better prognosis for patients with Ca bronchus? Clinical trials may be necessary to answer this question (Peckham, this volume).

Equipments similar to diagnostic CT scanners, but of lower specification, are available, and consideration is given to such alternative CT devices later in this volume. Whilst they may provide data for lung corrections some of them are unable to localise normal structures such as the kidneys, and it is doubtful if any of them can determine tumour extent to a greater degree than that achieved by conventional radiographs. Since even alternative CT devices are expensive, serious consideration should be given to other methods of imaging normal anatomy, such as ultrasound and the improvement of conventional radiology by methods such as digital radiography (Katragadda et al, 1979).

What other uses are there?

Whilst treatment charting and dose calculations have received the most attention, other applications of CT-assisted treatment planning require consideration. These are dealt with in part by other chapters.

1. Evaluation of treatment techniques

CT scans may be obtained with patients in different treatment positions, and the data used to evaluate various beam configurations. Comparison can be made based on considerations of integral dose, dose to critical organs, homogeneity through target volume, etc.

96

2. Three-dimensional distributions

Radiotherapy treatment planning usually considers a transverse plane through the centre of the treatment volume. It is important that the radiotherapist is aware of the isodose distribution in other planes. In the third dimension this can be represented by coronal and sagittal distributions, or many transverse sections throughout the target volume can be displayed.

Using the EMIPLAN equipment it is possible to plan a patient in the central plane of the treatment volume and then examine the corrected distribution in any number of off-axis planes.

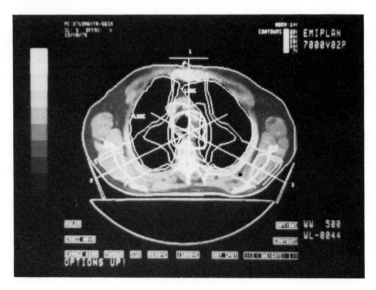

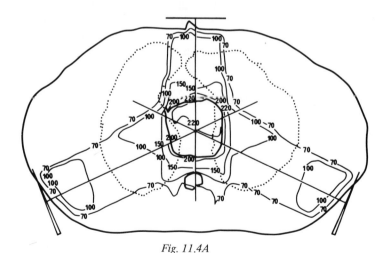

Fig. 11.4A

Fig. 11.4 Corrected isodose distribution for a three-field treatment of Ca oesophagus with 8 MeV photons. The distribution is given through the centre of the volume (Fig. 11.4A), 6 cm above (Fig. 11.4B) and 6 cm below (Fig. 11.4C).

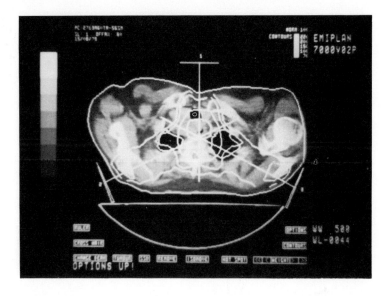

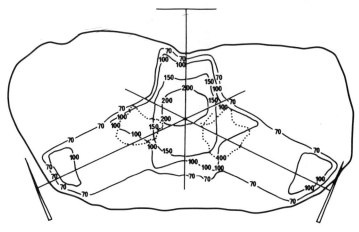

Fig. 11.4B

Figure 11.4 illustrates this facility with an example of Ca oesophagus. A 3-field 8 MeV photon distribution is shown, corrected for the effect of tissue inhomogeneities. Planes through the centre of the volume and 6 cm above and below have been calculated.

3. Breast treatments

The radiotherapeutic treatment of Ca breast occupies a considerable proportion of the work-load of most departments, and poses many specific problems. The prerequisite to any successful treatment method is careful planning and reproduc-

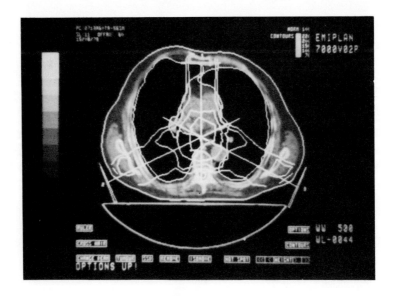

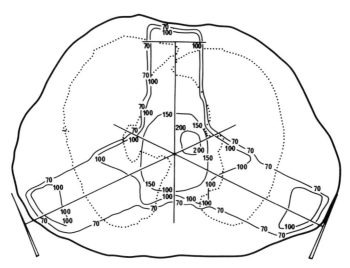

Fig. 11.4C

ibility of set-up. Unfortunately, the treatment positions currently used make it virtually impossible to scan a patient in the correct position on commercial CT scanners.

However, in Ca breast, the target volume is primarily decided by the anatomy rather than by tumour extent. Diagnostic quality scans are, therefore, of limited value, and if the scanner is only required for localisation then alternative CT devices may be used, where the image quality is poorer but the scan reconstruction area need not be so restricted. This may well prove to be the major application of such technology.

4. Plesiotherapy

The anatomical detail provided by CT in the treatment position can give useful information in planning an implant, and in ascertaining the position of the guides in after-loading techniques. It is unlikely that the spatial resolution of CT scanners in the longitudinal direction is sufficient for localisation prior to dose calculations.

What of the future?

The possibilities of using CT information for devising new techniques are at present unexplored. The improvements in localisation are likely to encourage trials of boost fields, and more accurate dosimetry (particularly with high energy electrons) could lead to increased use of mixed modality treatments.

We are already seeing the impact of quantitative monitoring of response on patient management, and such studies will, of course, lead to increased usage of CT scanners.

Of more immediate interest is the possibility of integrated planning.

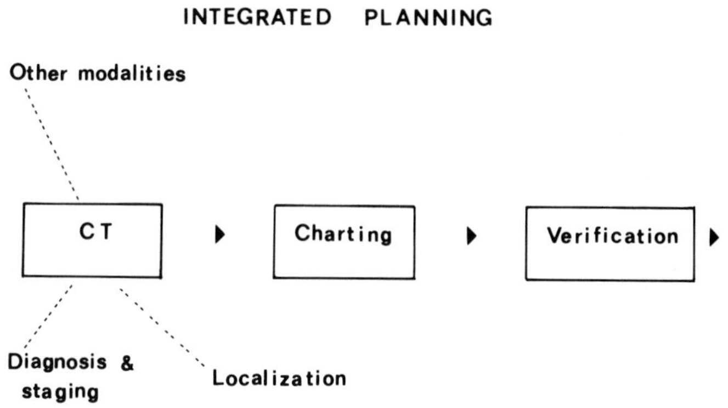

Fig. 11.5 Schematic diagram of integrated planning.

It is clear from earlier discussion that for selected patients the scanner is inherently capable of carrying out the localisation role of the radiotherapy simulator, but the mechanical accuracy of the scanner must be improved. It is now possible to obtain a scannogram (or 'scout-view') on the scanner itself (see Pullan, this volume), which can be used to relate external markings to internal anatomy and slice position. Such a concept deserves serious consideration since it would streamline the planning process for patients selected for CT-assisted treatment planning. The use of a simulator would still be advisable for verification of the field arrangement, and would of course be necessary in the planning of patients not undergoing CT scans.

Conclusions

The main strength of CT-assisted planning is in the localisation of the target volume, and good diagnostic images are required to determine tumour extent.

Patients who are to be treated with radical intent are therefore expected to benefit most from the technique. The full benefit of the improved localisation will not be achieved until the mechanical accuracy of the scanner is improved and advances made in techniques for positioning patients reproducibly. In the meantime, it must be appreciated that the CT scan obtained does not necessarily portray the anatomical situation during treatment.

Acknowledgements

We would like to record our appreciation for the help and advice of our many colleagues in the Departments of Physics, Radiotherapy and Radiology. Our especial thanks are due to Dr Neil Hodson and Dr Janet Husband for their help in assessing the impact of CT scans on radiotherapy plans. The studies on patient positioning were carried out by Mrs Ann Cattell, Mrs Jenny Sangway and Mrs Sue Unwin, with the assistance of Mr M. Heavens of EMI Medical Ltd.

References

Brizel H E, Livingstone P A, Grayson E V 1979 Radiotherapeutic applications of pelvic computed tomography. Journal of Computer Assisted Tomography 3(4): 453-466

Byhardt R W, Cox J D, Hamburg A, Liermann G 1978 Weekly localisation films and detection of field placement errors. International Journal of Radiation Oncology Biology and Physics 4: 881-887

Goitein M, Wittenberg J, Mendiondo M, Doucette J, Friedberg C, Ferruci J, Gunderson L, Linggood R, Shipley W V, Fineberg H W 1979 The value of CT scanning in radiation therapy treatment planning: a prospective study. International Journal of Oncology Biology and Physics 5: 1787-1798

Hobday P, Hodson N, Husband J, Parker R P, Macdonald J S 1979 Computed tomography applied to radiotherapy treatment planning: techniques and results. Radiology 133(2): 477-482

ICRU Report No 24 1976 International Commission on Radiation Units and Measurements Washington DC, USA

Katradagga C S, Fogel S R, Cohen G, Wagner L K, Morgan C, Handel S F, Amtey S R, Lester R G 1979 Digital radiography using a computed tomographic instrument. Radiology 133: 83-87

Macdonald J S, Parker R P, Husband J E, Hobday P A, Cattell A 1977 Change in treatment plans arising from CT scanning. Paper presented at 63rd meeting of Radiological Society of North America. Chicago, USA

Munzenrider J E, Pilepich M, Rene-Ferrero J B, Tchakarova I, Carter B L 1977 Use of body scanner in radiotherapy treatment planning. Cancer 40: 170-179

Parker R P, Hobday P A, Cassell K J 1979 The direct use of CT numbers in radiotherapy dosage calculations for inhomogeneous media. Physics Medicine Biology 24: 802-809

Parker R P, De Freitas L C, Cassell K J, Webb S, Hobday P A 1980 A method of implementing inhomogeneity corrections in radiotherapy treatment planning: comparison with experiment and Monte Carlo calculations. Journal Europeen de Radiotherapie (In press)

Parker R P 1980 The interface between a CT scanner and a treatment planning computer. Proc Workshop on CT scanners in radiotherapy in Europe, Geneva 1979. British Journal of Radiology Supplement 15 (In press)

Ragan D P, Perez C A 1978 Efficacy of CT-assisted two-dimensional treatment planning: analysis of 45 patients. American Journal of Roentgenology 131: 75-79

12. The application of CT to radiotherapy planning—head and neck

R. J. BERRY, WENDY JULIAN, N. NOSCOE and J. TWYDLE

Malignancies in head and neck sites are relatively infrequent in Europe and the western world. In the South Thames Metropolitan Regions, for which a good Cancer Registry allows reliable incidence data, during 1975 only 717 out of 25 125 (2.9 per cent) patients presenting with new malignancies for treatment had these tumours in head and neck sites. Of these, 78 per cent were treated by radiotherapy as part of their primary management, as compared to circa one-third of malignancies in all sites. At the Middlesex Hospital, during 1979 approximately 2700 patients were treated by radiotherapy and cytotoxic chemotherapy of whom circa 1500 presented for the first time. Of these, only 87 had malignancies in head and neck sites, and 12 of these were pituitary tumours, a special interest of our department.

Common medical practice in the treatment of head and neck tumours differs in the United Kingdom from that in other areas of the world (in particular North America) in that radiotherapy is regarded as the treatment of choice for the primary management of head and neck malignancies. Surgery is reserved for either the salvage of treatment failures or is used in a combined approach with planned surgery following preoperative radiotherapy. By contrast, in many parts of the world radical exenterative surgery is still the primary treatment for head and neck malignancies, and radiotherapy is largely reserved for the palliation of advanced disease or the treatment of surgical failures. At the Middlesex Hospital radiotherapy is employed as the primary treatment for attempting cure even in advanced disease in head and neck sites, with salvage surgery entirely reserved for treatment failures. Such failures, when they occur, present two major problems:

1. if the failure is within the high dose planned treatment volume, this must be regarded as a radiobiological failure. The proportion of such local failures will depend upon the choice of dose, the dose fractionation, and the accepted level of normal tissue damage which is considered to be 'tolerance'. In future it is hoped that many such failures may be dealt with by changes in dose fractionation once optimal patterns can be recognised for particular tumours, by the use of physical adjuncts such as hyperbaric oxygen or heat, by the use of densely ionising radiations such as fast neutrons whose effects are less dependent upon the presence or absence of oxygen, and less dependent on tissue repair, or by the use of pharmacological adjuncts such as selective radiosensitisers for hypoxic cells.

2. Failure to control primary tumours in head and neck sites is not uncommonly observed at the margins of the irradiated volume, and these must be regarded as

failure adequately to assess the spread of the tumour at the time of initial treatment planning. It is to these failures that improvements in tumour imaging are directed, as it is in the possible elimination of many of these failures that computed tomography has a significant potential contribution to make in reducing human misery. In head and neck sites more than any other, patient survival depends upon achieving permanent cessation of tumour growth at the primary site.

At the Middlesex Hospital, the EMI 5005 Body Scanner, situated in the Department of Radiotherapy and Oncology but operated jointly by a team comprising radiodiagnosticians, radiotherapists, medical physicists and radiographers, has been in operation since December 1977. In the period to 1 February 1980 a total of more than 3300 patients have been scanned, 118 had tumours in head and neck sites for which scans were undertaken specifically to aid planning their radiotherapy, while a further 57 had scans to assess the post-treatment responses of their tumours. In its present use, 55 per cent of all scans carried out on this general purpose machine are of the head, 45 per cent of the body. On average, 280 examinations are carried out per month on circa 150 patients, a total of over 2000 scans per month. During autumn 1979 we were privileged to instal the production prototype EMI Plan 7000 by which anatomical information from the CT Scanner can be transferred directly (by floppy disc) to a computerised radiotherapy planning system. This free-standing system, based on the Data General Eclipse computer, is not unlike the home-built system described by Sargood in a previous paper in this symposium. It uses the Data General RDOS operating system which, with compilers for FORTRAN and BASIC allows considerable programming flexibility, and is capable of operating in dual background/foreground modes. The installation of this sophisticated planning system and the arrival of the CT scanner at the Middlesex coincided with a project being carried out jointly by the Departments of Oncology and Physics as Applied to Medicine on optimising image quality and reducing patient dose in the use of xeroradiography and xerotomography for the localisation of head and neck tumours. We were therefore in the privileged position of having exceedingly high quality 'conventional' images against which to compare the new information provided by the computed tomographic scans (Bryant & Julian, 1978; Noscoe, 1980).

For some tumour sites in the head and neck, the well trained eye of the radiotherapist and his ENT surgeon colleague, aided by mirror or modern fibreoptic endoscopes and often supplemented by the ability to feel the tissues in question, give all the information necessary for assessing spread of tumour and for adequate planning of appropriate radiotherapy. These, supplemented by conventional radiographic imaging, make the beautiful images from computed tomography unnecessary in such a site as carcinoma of the larynx. Figure 12.1 shows the exceedingly high quality of the lateral xeroradiographic image used for treatment planning purposes. Antero-posterior xerotomograms offer a tremendous amount of information about the extent of disease in soft tissue, and because the xerotomogram visualises a rather deeper image due to its high resolution for the 'out of focus' portion, sufficient bony anatomical detail can be superimposed on the soft tissue image of interest to allow precise anatomical delimitation of the radiation treatment field. A comparison between a conventional film tomographic image of good diagnostic quality and a xerotomogram is shown in Figures 12.2B

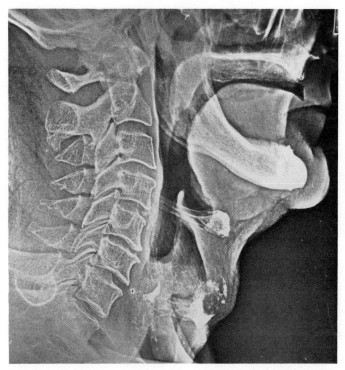

Fig. 12.1 Lateral xeroradiogram of patient with carcinoma of larynx. Note outstanding soft tissue detail in same image as bony anatomical landmarks.

and 12.2A respectively. The cost of such investigation is trivial in money terms compared with the cost of computed tomographic scans. In addition, in terms of radiation dose to the patient, the dose from complete xerotomographic examination is modest compared to the doses of up to 60 mGy (6 rads) per slice for high resolution computed tomographic scans in the head region. This radiation dose is, of course, of no importance in a region which is to receive high dose radiotherapy, but must be a consideration if repeated examinations are to be carried out during and after treatment to monitor tumour response.

For other head and neck sites, however, the assessment of extent of gross disease is less easy, even if one accepts the difficulty of predicting microscopic spread of tumour. For example, assessment of disease in the middle third of the tongue is often no more than an educated guess, while assessment of spread into the posterior third of the tongue must depend on such indirect evidence as the presence or absence of tethering. This is particularly difficult when prior surgery has made the normal anatomy difficult to unravel. In this site computed tomography has become an invaluable adjunct to the palpating finger in assessing such deep tumour extension, and indeed leads to hope of significant increases in tumour local control in this site, particularly when radiotherapy is given in conjunction with hyperbaric oxygen, with the hypoxic cell sensitisers, or given with densely ionising radiations such as fast neutrons.

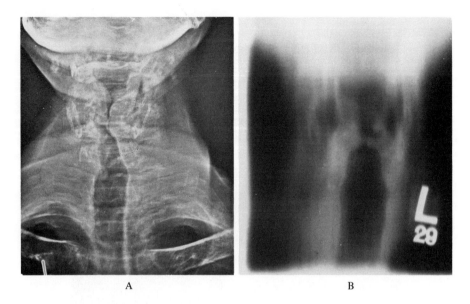

A   B

Fig. 12.2A AP xerotomogram of patient with carcinoma of larynx. Note soft tissue detail visible as well as bony landmarks for radiotherapy planning. Note image reversed left-right from conventional view.

Fig. 12.2B Conventional AP film tomogram of same patient. Note *no* visualisation of bony reference points.

One site where computed tomography has proved an outstanding advantage is in the treatment of tumours of the naxopharynx and paranasal sinuses. These tumours occur in areas where the position of the dose-limiting normal tissues, such as the lens of the eye and the brain stem, need to be known with a precision of only millimetres if unacceptable damage is not to be caused to them. Figure 12.3 shows

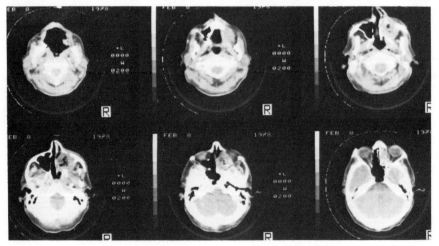

Fig. 12.3 CT scan of extensive squamous carcinoma of antrum. Note bony destruction and extension through anterior wall of antrum to skin.

a series of CT scans through an advanced squamous carcinoma of the antrum in which the bony destruction and extension of the tumour towards the skin shows the need for external build-up to achieve secondary charged particle equilibrium and hence uniform dose throughout the tumour volume. Conventional radiographic methods including xerotomography cannot resolve adequately the extent of such lesions because of the large number of complicating normal tissue shadows in conventional projections. Figure 12.4 shows the great usefulness of computed tomography in monitoring the change in tumour volume during and after treatment. In this case, the patient was a teenage girl with an embryonal rhabdomyosarcoma presenting as a fixed cervical node with only a small amount of visible disease found in the nasopharynx. The major problem in treatment planning was to attempt to spare the opposite eye. Although part of the tumour showed a dramatic initial response, it was clear during treatment that part of the tumour was continuing to grow and had extended across the middle line. This required extension of the radiation field, thus putting the opposite eye at risk. Later in treatment, when the tumour had clearly regressed, a shrinking field technique could again be used so that the total accumulated dose to the opposite eye would give little risk of loss of sight in this young patient. Adequate follow-up in this

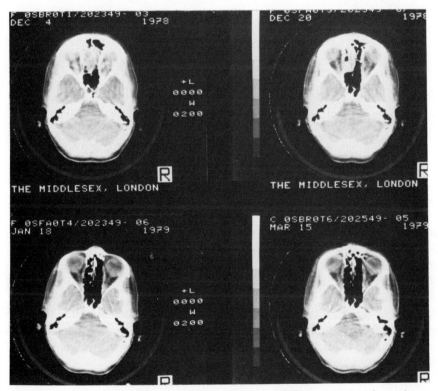

Fig. 12.4 Repeat CT scans of patient with embryonal rhabdomyosarcoma of nasopharynx. Note extension across mid-line during treatment (4 December 1978).
   Treatment field reduced after tumour shrinkage to mid-line to spare opposite eye (20 December 1978; 18 January 1979). Post treatment follow-up shows no local tumour recurrence (15 March 1979).

difficult site was only possible by the use of serial computed tomograms in specified planes, and although in spite of adjuvant cytotoxic therapy she developed disseminated disease and died at one year, the primary site remained disease-free.

We are only just beginning to appreciate the value of direct superimposition of anatomical information from the CT scan and the computed treatment plan using the EMI Plan System 7000. Figure 12.5 shows the hard copy print-out of such a plan. We have shown that it is technically possible without significant loss of

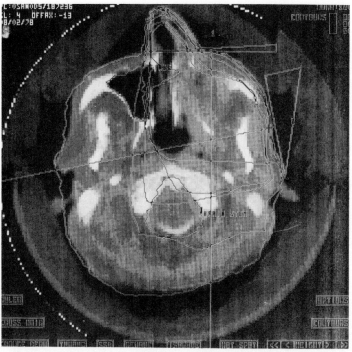

Fig. 12.5 Hard copy print-out of radiotherapy treatment plan from EMI Plan 7000 super-imposed on CT scan; this is the same patient as shown in Figure 12.3.

diagnostic detail to scan the patient within a Darvic shell, which would be used for holding the patient immobile during fractionated treatment. Thus, the position of not only the tumour but the limiting normal tissues can be reproduced to millimetre accuracy, allowing us to take advantage of the additional anatomical information provided by the CT scan. Input to the planning system is by keyboard, light pen or graphical tablet and allows great flexibility. Compensation for tissue heterogeneity can be made either using bulk volume corrections for defined areas or, demanding additional computational time but still within acceptable real time limits, using pixel by pixel correction based on EMI numbers.

With over two years experience of the use of CT scanning in head and neck tumours we find it to be a most useful adjunct to both the initial assessment of tumour volume and for monitoring changes in tumour volume during treatment for those head and neck sites where modern conventional radiographic techniques (including xeroradiography and xerotomography) are unhelpful. A specific advantage is the ability to scan the patient within the immobilising shell which will be used for actual treatment and the possibility of direct transfer of anatomical information from the scan to the EMI Plan computerised planning system. The cost in both money terms and radiation dose of computed tomography is high, but it is totally justified when patient survival depends upon achieving tumour local control and when alternative imaging techniques fail to demonstrate adequately the extent of tumour, and the exact position of limiting normal structures.

References

Bryant T H E, Julian W 1978 Reduction of radiation doses in patients in xeroradiography. British Journal of Radiology 51: 974-980

N J Noscoe 1980 Xerotomography of the larynx – an aid to radiotherapy planning. (Submitted to Radiography)

South Thames Cancer Registry 1975 Evidence to the London Health Care Consortium Working Party on Radiotherapy and Oncology 1979 p 4

13. Clinical value of CT in thoracic treatment planning

T. G. LANDBERG, T. R. MÖLLER and I-L LAMM

Computed tomography is useful at different stages of the radiotherapy procedure. Firstly, it gives diagnostic information about the tumour which is essential for the definition of the target volume. CT also provides information on patient outline(s), borders of the target volume(s) and other internal structures of interest. For the physical dose planning, CT gives qualitative information on patient outline and internal organs and furthermore has the capability of giving quantitative information on tissue properties which can be used for inhomogeneity corrections to the dose distribution. CT is also useful for the follow up during and after treatment.

Optimisation

One of the ways to improve the results of radiotherapy is to improve the distribution of absorbed dose in the target volume and in other tissues, aiming at an increased therapeutic ratio. This procedure of optimisation in radiotherapy should include not only the physical treatment planning but also the other steps in the total procedure, namely the diagnostic examination, the staging, the localisation for treatment planning, the execution of treatment and the follow up after therapy. Since a uniform tumour dose with a negligible dose to uninvolved tissues can rarely be achieved, it is necessary to evaluate the absorbed dose distribution for the target volume and other tissues of interest for different treatment techniques. There are different criteria for optimisation of the physical dose plan, some often reported are listed in Table 13.1. In addition, personal preference or judgement is often made for the 'best' distribution. Computers can be used to compare differ-

Table 13.1 Criteria for optimsation of dose distributions

1. The minimum target(s) absorbed dose(s) should be the prescribed target dose.

2. The absorbed dose in the target volume should be as homogeneous as possible.

3. The absorbed dose to organs at risk should be as low as possible, and at least below an accepted limit.

4. The integral dose should be as low as possible.

5. The treatment should be as simple as possible in order to minimize technical errors.

6. The treatment should be technically feasible.

ent plans and the selection of the optimum plan is performed by examining a limited number of quantifiable parameters. To aid this choice the treatment planning system should at least supply information about maximum, minimum, mean, median and modal target absorbed dose as well as absorbed dose anywhere in the section. For optimisation by personal judgement, an absorbed dose profile for the target area may be useful (Fig. 13.1). Of course, sophistication of

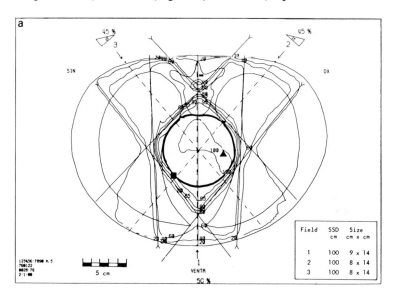

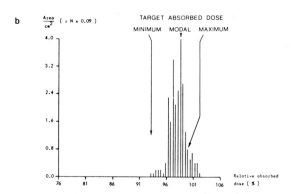

Fig. 13.1 Computerised calculation of the absorbed dose distribution (8 MV X-rays) for a patient with carcinoma of the oesophagus. (a) dose distribution in the transverse section. (b) histogram to demonstrate the distribution of absorbed dose in the target area. For details see ICRU Report 29 (1978) (By kind permission from ICRU Washington D.C.)

methodology should include all steps in the whole procedure in order to achieve the best total results. Without doubt, the localisation procedure for dose planning, including the representation of target volume(s), organs at risk, and tissue hetero-geneities is often recognised to be a very weak link. It appears that CT will prove very useful in improving this part of the whole treatment procedure. Furthermore, CT offers a unique possibility to evaluate the physical properties of the various tissues in the irradiated volume.

Body sections for dose planning

A uniform dose distribution can rarely be achieved in the target volume and it is, therefore, necessary to evaluate the spatial absorbed dose distribution throughout the entire volume. Such an evaluation could be made in principle by considering the dose distribution in a set of parallel transverse sections sufficiently close to each other, e.g. the distance between two sections being equal to the distance between the lattice points of the dose planning system. However, for practical reasons, only a limited number of sections can be evaluated. These sections may be selected in the following way (ICRU Report 29, 1978) (Fig. 13.2). The part of the patient

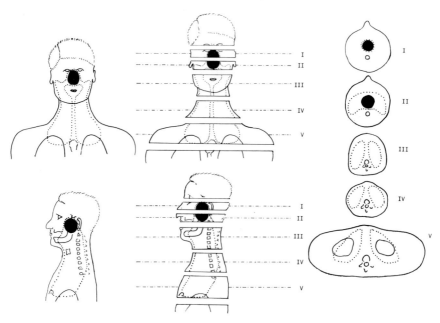

Fig. 13.2 Example of multiple sections for dose-planning in a patient with carcinoma of the nasopharynx. For details, see ICRU Report 29 (1978). (By kind permission from ICRU Washington DC)

containing the target volume and relevant anatomical structures is considered to consist of a stack of slices, the thickness of them being chosen so that in each slice the following conditions are fulfilled:

    a. No important variations occur in the external contour.

    b. No important variations occur in the topography of the relevant internal structures: size, shape and location of the target volume, organs at risk, tissue heterogeneities, etc.

    c. No important variations are expected in the dose distribution that are relevant to the treatment plan. For each slice a section is chosen (Fig. 13.2) on which the extreme borders of the target volume, the organs at risk, the tissue heterogeneities and the reference points in that slice are projected perpendicularly. The sections then display all the relevant structures and the part of the target volume which is located within the slice now appears as a target area. In many simple situations, e.g. carcinoma of the urinary bladder, consideration is given only to one section, whereas in other situations several sections will have to be considered in order to give an adequate picture of the whole absorbed dose distribution. This is particularly true for the thoracic region (Fig. 13.3), where at different levels the

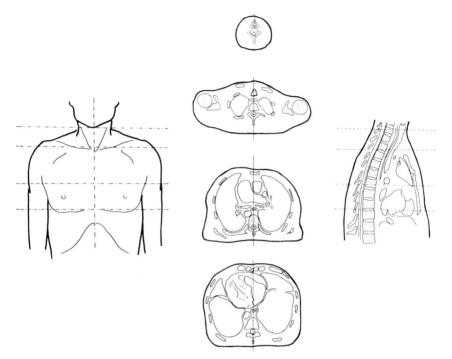

Fig. 13.3 Example of 4 transverse and one sagittal section used for the planning of treatment of a patient with a thoracic tumour.

body contour and internal topography as well as the distribution of tissue heterogeneities varies greatly and often four or even more sections will have to be used for dose planning. The dose distribution is usually calculated in the transverse section, but sagittal (Fig. 13.3) as well as oblique or even tilted sections may be usefully examined. It should be mentioned that for some special treatment techniques, e.g. dynamic treatment, the number of required sections may be very large and approach a true three-dimensional situation. When using CT for obtaining anatomical information for the physical dose planning, it is essential that the patient is examined in the treatment position using all devices that will be used during treatment, e.g. casts of different kinds and any bolus material. In general, only one treatment position should be used, since change of posture may result in change in external contour, tilting of the vertical axis through the patient, and shift of internal structures. It is generally very difficult to add dose distributions obtained with different treatment positions.

Special tomographic situations

Lymphoma

The contribution of CT to the treatment of lymphomas was reported by Pilepich et al (1978) for 42 chest examinations. The finding at CT of mediastinal expansion and extension into the lung tissue from the hila had, with the standard treatment techniques in the department, no implications whereas spread along the chest wall anteriorly (seen in all types of lymphoma) and posteriorly (seen in non-Hodgkin's lymphomas) had therapeutic implications in 9 out of 15 patients. Mink et al (1978) reported CT of the anterior mediastinum in patients with myasthenia gravis and suspected thymoma to yield significant information in 3 out of 5 cases (e.g. pleural spread).

Bronchogenic carcinoma

The value of CT in radiotherapeutic management of lung cancer has been the subject of several reports. Emami et al (1978) reported on 48 patients in whom a better delineation of the tumour extent was seen in 35 (73 per cent) and a change in assessment of size of the lesion was done in 25 (52 per cent). A change in stage due to CT findings was made in 21 (43 per cent) patients. Demonstration of inadequacy of coverage was done in 16/45 (33 per cent) and changes in the volume of normal tissues irradiated could be done in 22/45 (48 per cent). Unsuspected areas of involvement were seen in 32 of the 48 patients (67 per cent) and CT was judged totally as essential for treatment planning in 26 out of 46 evaluated patients (57 per cent). In a similar study Hodson et al (1979) compared CT with conventional planning in 45 patients and found tumour coverage with conventional methods to be inadequate in 12 (26 per cent) and marginal in 6 (13 per cent). Using CT the target volume increased in 5 (11 per cent), reduced in 1 (2 per cent) and moved in 7 (15 per cent). A discrepancy in body contour of at least 1.5 cm was seen in 9 (20 per cent). In 15 patients (33 per cent) the plans were altered after CT information had been obtained.

Mammary carcinoma

Munzenrider et al (1977) found CT data essential for treatment planning of thoracic tumours in 14 patients, helpful in 4 and not necessary in 3. For the chest wall/breast the corresponding figures were 2, 2 and 0. Munzenrider et al (1979) recommended routine determinations of chest wall thickness in patients planned for electron beam treatment, in obese patients and in patients treated with tangential photon techniques to avoid under-dosage to the internal mammary nodes.

Tissue heterogeneities

CT gives information on the radiation attenuating properties of different tissues and thus allows for a defined correction for tissue heterogeneity from the first treatment session. For the thoracic region the presence of gas in the air passages and lungs and the mineral bone in the vertebral bodies should be taken into account, whereas the ribs are usually ignored in this connection. The lungs present the greatest problem. Even with a simple AP-PA treatment with high energy photons the difference in absorbed dose distribution with and without correction for lung tissue is pronounced and may for the hilar regions amount to 30 per cent. Also for electrons (Fig. 13.4) this effect may be significant and eliminate some of the advantages with this type of radiation.

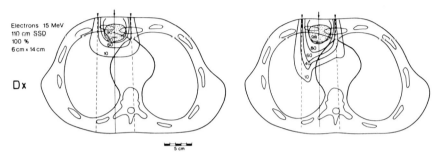

Fig. 13.4 Treatment of the internal mammary nodes with electrons (15 MeV). Left: without correction for tissue heterogeneity. Right: corrected for lung tissue. From ICRU Report 29 (1978) (By kind permission from ICRU Washington DC)

Fullerton et al (1978) studied the oesophageal absorbed dose in 3 patients using measurements of absorbed dose in the oesophagus during treatment as the reference (100 per cent). Using a 'standard' technique and assuming the lung density to be $= 0.33$, the corresponding dose values were 92-103 per cent and using a plan based on the CT examination, the values were 99-103 per cent. Sternick et al (1977) compared several plans for a patient with carcinoma of the oesophagus, using on one hand transverse axial tomography and ultrasonic scanning and on the other hand CT. Average tissue densities and the CT numbers were used, respectively. The average deviation between treatment plans calculated for the conventional and for the CT method was 10.4 per cent and 7.1 per cent for cobalt-60 gamma rays and for 6 MV photons respectively for the target volume. Surprisingly, even larger differences were found for the absorbed dose values for the spinal cord (27.1 per cent and 23.7 per cent respectively).

Estimation of impact on dose distribution

An example is given in Figure 13.5 of the effects of (1) the lack of corrections for tissue heterogeneities, (2) incorrect outer contour and (3) incorrect inner topography of the lungs, on evaluation of absorbed dose in the target volume, lungs and spinal cord, for a patient with carcinoma of the oesophagus treated with the same technique as shown in Figure 13.1. The values were calculated for a particular patient of standard shape and size. The lung correction factors were based on in vivo measurements of absorbed dose in the oesophagus during treatment, the 'effective bone density' being 1.3 in relation to muscle tissue. For the example chosen, lack of correction for tissue heterogeneity gave a calculated target absorbed dose of 0.85 of the correct value, whereas an error of 1.5 cm in contours gave values between 0.92 and 0.90. For the lung tissue lack of correction

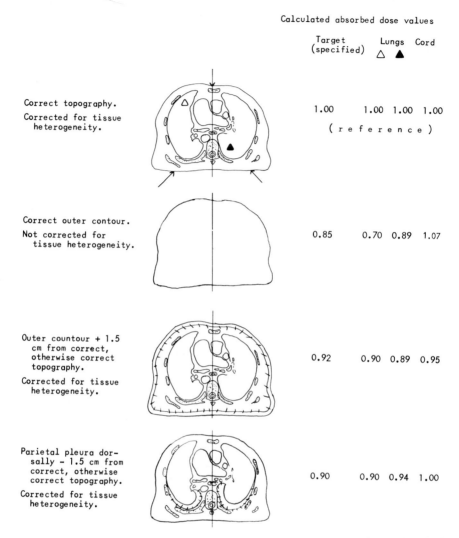

Calculated absorbed dose values

	Target (specified)	Lungs △	▲	Cord

Correct topography.
Corrected for tissue heterogeneity.

1.00   1.00 1.00 1.00

(r e f e r e n c e)

Correct outer contour.
Not corrected for tissue heterogeneity.

0.85   0.70 0.89 1.07

Outer countour + 1.5 cm from correct, otherwise correct topography.
Corrected for tissue heterogeneity.

0.92   0.90 0.89 0.95

Parietal pleura dorsally - 1.5 cm from correct, otherwise correct topography.
Corrected for tissue heterogeneity.

0.90   0.90 0.94 1.00

Fig 13.5 Effects of tissue heterogeneity and proper evaluation of topography on the calculation of absorbed dose in the target area and organs at risk for a patient with carcinoma of the oesophagus. Same treatment technique as shown in Figure 13.1 for a prone patient.

for heterogeneity underestimated grossly the absorbed dose (0.70-0.89 of the true values). An error of 1.5 cm in contours gave values of lung absorbed dose of 0.89-0.94 of the true values. The spinal cord dose was less influenced by errors, lack of heterogeneity correction (bone) giving the false value 1.07, and incorrect outer contour giving a value for cord dose of 0.95 of the correct value. The deviations in these examples of calculated absorbed dose from the true ones may well represent relevant clinical situations. They may exceed the limit ± 5 per cent, which has been recognised to result in changes in cure rate and incidence of radiation side effects (ICRU Report 24, 1976). In the chest region the deviations often tend to be in the directions towards overdosage, due to the presence of lung tissue, which may be particularly harmful if treatment is brought up towards normal connective tissue tolerance (e.g. boost therapy). On the other hand, the presence of mineral bone in the vertebral column may introduce a risk of underdosage in mediastinal structures, especially with standard AP-PA treatment techniques.

Ragan & Perez (1978) presented a method for quantitatively assessing the impact of CT-assisted treatment planning. Non-uniformity and local efficiency of dose delivered were compared without and with the utilisation of CT information. In 31 of the 45 patients, plans were improved with the use of CT information. The areas in which the greatest gains were made were the brain, lung (3 patients) and retroperitoneum.

Follow up

Since the treatment plan obviously should only be used as long as it is valid, a careful follow up during treatment is mandatory. Simple measures, such as control of the patient's weight or repeat measurements of absorbed dose in or at the patient, are helpful but may not give reliable information about changes in the section's outline and contents. Repeat CT during treatment will then be recommended.

Technical and financial aspects

Desirable properties of a CT scanner when used for planning radiation treatment of thoracic tumours

Apparently a CT scanner, when used for treatment planning purposes, will have to fulfil certain requirements. These may not all be relevant to a purely diagnostic scanner. Table 13.2 lists some of the requirements that may be asked for when

Table 13.2 Some specific desirable properties of a CT scanner when used for planning treatment of thoracic tumours. Modified after Goitein (1979)

1. Excellent spatial and absorbtion coefficient resolution, being of the order of 7 lines pairs per centimeter.

2. Capability of scanning a large number (about 60) of relatively thin (5 mm or less) sections continuously at a rate of one section per 10 seconds. High anode and X-ray tube housing cooling rates and high geometric and photons conversion efficiencies of the detectors.

3. Capacity to generate and AP and a lateral 'plain film' ('scout view') referenced to scan sections.

4. Large mechanical aperture (diameter 60 cm) and large (at least 50 cm) diameter of reconstruction.

5. Sagittal and coronal display capabilities. Ability to construct oblique sections and tilted (about 0-15 degrees) sections.

6. Possibility to duplicate a purely diagnostic scan.

defining the properties of a CT scanner for therapy planning purposes. It may be added that the scanner should be able to connect directly to the treatment planning system in order to minimise potential errors, e.g. those connected with the transferral of digital information to analogue and back again to digital.

Cost-benefit considerations

The costs of CT are an obstacle to its widespread use in radiation treatment planning. It has been estimated (Stewart, 1977) that an increase of only 3-4 per cent in cure rate would warrant economically the routine use of two therapy-related CT scans in 2/3 of all patients who receive radiotherapy. Since patients who succumb to bronchogenic carcinoma or carcinoma of the oesophagus, 11 per cent and 59 per cent respectively, do so as a result of uncontrolled primary tumour (Suit, 1976), the use of CT in these diseases for treatment planning may well be warranted. For lymphomas the case may be somewhat different with respect to tumour healing, since treatment of recurrent disease is often effective though, admittedly, less often so than primary treatment. However, because of the large volumes that are irradiated in lymphomas, a substantial gain may be made with respect to normal tissue radiation reactions through the use of CT.

References

Emami B, Melo A, Carter B L, Munzenrider J E, Piro A J 1978 The value of computed tomography in radiotherapeutic management of lung cancer. International Journal of Radiation Oncology Biology and Physics 4 (suppl. 2); 200

Fullerton G D, Sewchand W, Payne T, Levitt S H 1978 CT determination of parameters for inhomogeneity corrections in radiation therapy of the oesophagus. Radiology 126: 167-171

Goitein M 1979 Computed tomography in planning radiation therapy. International Journal of Radiation Oncology Biology and Physics 5: 445-447

Hodson N J, Husband J, Hobday P 1979 Computed tomography and treatment planning – techniques and clinical implications. Proc. Int. Symp., Fundamentals in technical progress, Liege, May 11-12 1979. Volume II, 9. 1-19

ICRU Report 24 1976 Determination of absorbed dose in a patient irradiated by beams of X or gamma rays in radiotherapy procedures. ICRU, International Commission on radiation units and measurements, Washington D.C.

ICRU Report 29 1978 Dose specification for reporting external beam therapy with photons and electrons ICRU, International Commission on radiation units and measurements, Washington D.C.

Mink J H, Marshall E B, Sukov R, Herrmann Ch Jr, Winter J, Sample W F, Mulder D 1978 Computed tomography of the anterior mediastinum in patients with myastenia gravis and suspect thymoma. American Journal of Roentgenology 130: 239-246

Munzenrider J E, Pilepich M, Rene-Ferrero J B, Tchakarova I, Carter B L, 1977 Use of body scanner in radiotherapy treatment planning. Cancer 40: 170-179

Munzenrider J E, Tchakarova I, Castro M, Carter B 1979 Computerised body tomography in breast cancer. I. Internal mammary nodes and radiation treatment planning. Cancer 43: 137-150

Pilepich M V, Rene J B, Munzenrider J E, Carter B L 1978 Contribution of computed tomography to the treatment of lymphomas. American Journal of Roentgenology 131: 69-73

Ragan D P, Perez C A 1978 Efficacy of CT-assisted two-dimensional treatment planning: analysis of 45 patients. American Journal of Roentgenology 131: 75-79

Sternick E S, Lane F W, Curran B 1977 Comparison of computed tomography and conventional transverse axial tomography in radiotherapy treatment planning. Radiology 124: 835-836

Stewart J R 1977 Computed tomography and the quality of radiation therapy. American Journal of Roentgenology 129: 943-944

Suit H D 1970 Introduction – Statement of the problem pertaining to the effect of dose fractionation and total treatment time on response of tissue to x-irradiation. In: Time and dose relationships in radiation biology as applied to radiation therapy. Proc. NCI-AEC Conf., September, 1969. Brookhaven Natl. Lab. Report BNL 50203 (C57), 1970

14. A critical appraisal of the value of CT to the radiotherapist—the abdomen

J. E. MUNZENRIDER, L. VERHEY and J. DOUCETTE

Introduction

Delivering radical radiotherapy to abdominal malignancies has been hampered by several factors: the relative radioresistance of most intra-abdominal tumors, especially adenocarcinomas of the GI tract, biliary system, pancreas, and kidneys; the radiosensitivity of adjacent normal structures (stomach, small and large intestine, liver, kidneys, spinal cord) and the difficulty in determining the extent of abdominal tumors and their relation to normal radiosensitive intra- and retro-peritoneal structures for accurate radiation treatment planning.

Abdominal imaging

Conventional abdominal imaging techniques, including GI procedures, arterio-graphy, and radionuclide scans, are limited in their ability to delineate tumor extent. Some tumors, particularly those of the pancreas and liver, and enlarged para-aortic nodes, can be visualised by B-mode ultrasound. However, the localation of dose-limiting abdominal organs relative to tumors defined by these techniques can only be approximated from such studies.

The revolutionary nature of computerised tomography has been universally and justifiably recognised by the recent decision of the Nobel committee to award the 1979 Nobel Prize in Medicine jointly to Hounsfield and Cormack, for their independent contributions to the development of that technique. Physicians in general and radiotherapists in particular are responding to the challenge of appreciating the potential and limitations of this new technique, and defining criteria for its application in clinical practice. Early experience with body scanners has demonstrated that the technique was capable of identifying abdominal lymph node masses, retroperitoneal tumors, and pancreatic disease, frequently more completely than other methods, or where other methods had failed to delineate such lesions. Kreel (1977) has described technical aspects of the general purpose scanner (one capable of scanning any part of the body including the head), listed clinical applications of the unit and summarised results obtained in studying particular organs and lesions, including retroperitoneal tumors and lymph nodes, the pancreas, liver and kidneys, and the appearance of peritoneal infiltration and ascites. He also has described general aspects of patient preparation and positioning, as well as techniques for localisation of a particular scan section relative to bony (vertebral) landmarks. More recently, Wittenberg & Ferrucci (1978) have reviewed experience gained with the first two generations of body scanners in abdominal imaging, concluding that the morphological representation of abdominal solid tumors provided by computerised body tomography (CT) is not only superior to all other imaging techniques, but is also non-invasive and associated with a relatively low level of radiation exposure to the patient. These two factors were thought to make it preferable to angiography in situations where equivalent information could be obtained from either technique. However, they point out that radionuclide scans and ultrasonography are also non-invasive, the latter gives no patient radiation exposure, and furnishes saggital as well as transverse images. Thus, while several non-invasive imaging techniques are available to study abdominal tumors, there is still insufficient data to define appropriate imaging protocols for a given clinical situation.

Tissue diagnosis and follow-up

The use of CT-guided fine needle aspiration of abdominal and pelvic tumors has been reviewed by Ferrucci & Wittenberg (1978), who themselves obtained positive cytology from 25 patients subsequently confirmed by surgically obtained biopsy. The utility of CT in the clinical follow up of abdominal malignancy has been alluded to by Kreel (1977), Munzenrider et al (1977) and Pilepich et al (1978). Lee and associates (1978) have reviewed 132 scans in 101 previously scanned patients with known or suspected abdominal or pelvic masses; 63 of the patients had known malignancy. Their data demonstrates that CT is quite useful in following progression or regression of tumor masses after treatment. Serial scans alone aided in defining mass status or confirming absence of mass in 71 per cent of cases. The scan provided new information in 16 per cent of cases, and was not helpful or was misleading in only 2 per cent and 6 per cent of cases, respectively. Serial scans were helpful in assessing tumor status in 96 per cent of lymphoma patients, 90 per cent of pancreatic cases, and 72 per cent of patients with retroperitoneal disease.

CT has proven to be of major significance in imaging abdominal tumors, has aided in identifying their histological type by guiding percutaneous aspiration biopsy, and has been of value in following patients with abdominal tumors following treatment.

Computerised tomography in radiation treatment planning

Early clinical efforts with CT were directed towards defining its utility as an imaging technique, and in determining which categories of patients might benefit from its application. It soon became apparent that the technique had great potential for radiotherapy treatment planning, since the scan provided a transverse body contour containing an exact image of the tumor and of the relationship of the tumor volume to dose-limiting normal tissues.

Tufts-New England Medical Center Study

Recognising that radiotherapy depends heavily on imaging techniques for tumor diagnosis, for determination of tumor extent, and for localising tumors for treatment planning to deliver an adequate dose to the target volume without exceeding the tolerance of uninvolved adjacent normal tissues, Munzenrider et al (1977) acknowledged the responsibility of the radiation therapist to appreciate the potential and limitations of the technique, and reviewed the literature relating to tumor imaging and radiotherapy treatment planning with CT. They also retrospectively analysed scans of 98 radiotherapy patients who had been studied with CT at the Tufts-New England Medical Center, to determine what contribution the scan made to management of those patients. Scans were available for treatment planning in 25 abdominal patients and in 50 with non-abdominal sites. Coverage of the scan-defined tumor volume would not have been adequate in 60 per cent of abdominal patients, and in 40 per cent of patients with tumors at other sites, if only non-CT data had been employed for treatment planning. Unsuspected areas of involvement were seen in 59 per cent of abdominal and in only 33 per cent of non-abdominal scans. A reduction in the volume of normal tissue irradiated was made possible with CT data in 44 per cent of abdominal patients and in only 16 per cent of patients being planned for treatment at other sites. When CT data was incorporated, a change in the total volume irradiated occurred in 56 per cent of abdominal patients, compared with 40 per cent of non-abdominal patients. The scan was deemed essential for treatment planning in 64 per cent of abdominal patients and in 50 per cent of the patients being planned for treatment to non-abdominal sites. Thus, in planning treatment to abdominal sites, availability of CT data impacted significantly on the total volume treated, the volume of normal tissue irradiated, and the degree of adequacy of tumor coverage. The scan was judged essential for treatment planning in almost two-thirds of abdominal patients studied. Contributions of the scan to evaluation of and treatment planning in the abdominal patients and patients with non-abdominal sites are summarised in Table 14.1.

Table 14.1 Contribution of scan to treatment planning: Tufts-New England Medical Center Study

Contribution of scan	Abdomen 25 patients %	Other sites 50 patients %
Tumor coverage not adequate	60	40
Unsuspected involvement seen	59	33
Normal tissue volume reduced	44	16
Treatment volume changed	56	40
Essential for planning	64	50

Massachusetts General Hospital Study

In a similarly structured but prospective study, Goitein et al (1979), have assessed the value of CT in treatment planning for 77 patients, 14 of whom had abdominal tumors. Treatment was planned with all available patient data before CT scan was performed, then re-planned utilising CT data. Overall, 40 of the 77 patients (52 per cent) had some change in their treatment plan as a result of the scan findings. Eighty-six per cent of abdominal patients had a change in plan due to CT findings, compared to 44 per cent of the non-abdominal patients studied. Most patients received treatment to a large volume initially, followed by a 'boost' to the demonstrable tumor mass itself. Treatment plans were evaluated for tumor coverage, with a tumor 'miss' occurring if a portion of the target volume lay outside the edge of one or more of the treatment portals. Using these definitions, a 'miss' would have occurred with the large volume treatment in 14 per cent of abdominal patients and in 13 per cent of the non-abdominal group. A 'miss' was observed for the boost portion of the treatment in 43 per cent of abdominal patients and in only 18 per cent of the others. The scan was of major significance for treatment planning in 64 per cent of abdominal patients and in only 30 per cent of patients with non-abdominal sites. The scan was also valuable in selecting patient position for treatment with important changes in normal tissue coverage being produced by treating in a particular position suggested by the scan. The reproducibility of anatomic relationships defined by CT had been verified with repeat scans in situations where critical normal tissue tolerances were involved, or where post-surgical changes were suspected to have occurred. Contributions of the scan to treatment planning in these patients are summarised in Table 14.2.

Table 14.2 Contribution of scan to treatment planning: Massachusetts General Hospital Study

Contribution of scan	Abdomen 14 patients %	Other sites 63 patients %
Change in plan	86	44
'Miss'		
Large volume	14	13
Boost	43	18
Major significance	64	30

Royal Marsden Hospital Study

Techniques and results of the application of CT to radiotherapy treatment planning have also been recently described by Hobday and associates (1979). Two requirements for the scan to be of significance in treatment planning were outlined: that it provide good diagnostic information about the tumor and its relationship to surrounding structures, and that it furnish cross sectional data relevant to the proposed treatment volume, including visual data relating to body contour and the location of internal structures as well as quantitative data for tissue hetero-geneity corrections. A protocol for comparing treatment plans incorporating CT data with those done with conventional techniques was applied to 123 patients planned for radical treatment. Special precautions were taken to assure that scan conditions simulated those that would exist during radiotherapy. CT data was transferred directly from the scanner to the treatment planning computer, and quantitative CT data was employed directly for inhomogeneity corrections. Respiration was noted to degrade the diagnostic image more significantly in the abdomen, relative to the pelvis and the thorax, with respiratory motion contribut-ing to poor scan quality in 37 per cent of abdominal scans, and in only 12 per cent of pelvic and thoracic scans. Changes in the body contour due to respiration were observed in 32 per cent of abdominal patients and in only 6 per cent of non-abdominal patients. In two cases, the treatment volume moved on and off the tumor with movement of the anterior abdominal wall during respiration. Ten pancreatic and 9 retroperitoneal tumors were studied: tumor coverage was inadequate in 58 per cent of these abdominal patients, but in only 19 per cent of non-abdominal patients studied.

Treatment volume was altered in 68 per cent of abdominal patients, and in only 22 per cent of pelvic and thoracic patients. Overall, availability of CT data produced a change in 79 per cent of the abdominal patients, and in only 31 per cent of pelvic and thoracic patients. Kidney position for blocking purposes was incorrect in 56 per cent of 9 patients when renal position from the scan was compared with that from other studies. Spinal cord position from conventional studies was incorrect in 3 of 30 thoracic patients studied, a noteworthy figure, since a significant constraint in treatment planning for upper abdominal tumors, including those of the pancreas and stomach, and for para aortic nodes is to avoid exceeding spinal cord tolerance. It was concluded that in this selected group of patients being planned for radical radiotherapy, CT scanning had played a significant role in treatment planning, especially in patients with abdominal tumors. Neither internal anatomy nor tumor was observed to move transversely with respiration. Advantages of direct transfer of CT data from scanner to treatment planning computer were discussed, especially freedom from distortion of the CT image, since distortion may occur when indirect photographic techniques are employed for treatment planning purposes. Contributions of the scan to treatment planning in abdominal and in non-abdominal patients are summarised in Table 14.3.

Table 14.3 Contribution of scan to treatment planning: Royal Marsden Hospital Study

Contribution of scan	Abdomen 19 patients %	Other sites 104 patients %
Change in body contour with respiration	32	6
Tumor coverage not adequate	58	19
Treatment volume changed	68	22
Total change in treatment	79	31
Kidney position incorrect[a]	56	
Spinal cord position incorrect[b]		10

[a] 9 patients
[b] 30 thoracic patients

Comparison of results of these three studies

These three studies on the utility of CT in abdominal tumors were structured differently and came from 3 different institutions with varying treatment policies, conventional planning facilities and computer expertise. Their remarkably similar conclusions are summarised and compared in Table 14.4. Inadequate tumor cover-

Table 14.4 Summary: contribution of scan to abdominal treatment planning in
three studies

Contribution of scan	Tufts Study 25 patients %	MGH Study 14 patients %	Royal Marsden Study 19 patients %
Tumor coverage inadequate	60	57[a]	53
Treatment volume changed	56		68
Change in plan		86	79
'Essential'	64		
'Major significance'		64	

[a] 14% 'Miss' large field and 43 'Miss' boost field

age was seen in 60 per cent, 57 per cent, and 53 per cent of abdominal patients
studied. Similar percentages of patients had a change in treatment volume and
plan. The scan was judged 'essential' and of 'major significance' in an identical
64 per cent of 25 patients studied by Munzenrider et al (1977) and of 14 patients
studied by Goitein et al (1979).

The results of these studies clearly demonstrate the inherent value of the scan
in providing valuable information regarding abdominal tumors, and indicate the
gross inadequacy of conventional techniques in localising abdominal tumors for
radiotherapy treatment planning.

Limitations and pitfalls in use of CT for treatment planning

Remarkable improvement in imaging abdominal tumors for radiotherapy treatment
planning with CT has been demonstrated in the three studies cited above.
However, there are significant limitations to the utilisation of CT data in
treatment planning; numerous pitfalls await the unwary treatment planner who
employs this revolutionary new tool. These limitations and pitfalls will be discussed
in detail below.

Significant difficulties exist in *registering* the level of the transverse scan showing
the tumor and surrounding normal structures to external or internal landmarks
which may be employed for treatment simulation and verification: special
techniques must be employed to register the patient in a knowable and accurate
way so that transverse image data may be accurately employed to localise the
tumor and adjacent normal organs in the saggital and coronal planes. Significant
variation in organ and/or tumor position may occur with changes in *patient
position,* making hazardous or potentially disastrous the localisation of structures
of interest on a scan taken in one position for treatment planning in another
position. *Patient immobilisation* in a reproducible fashion, both for scanning and
for treatment simulation and execution, may be necessary, especially if non-
supine techniques are employed, either to shift normal structures out of the
treatment volume or because of therapy unit constraints in terms of beam
direction, etc. *Involuntary patient motion* during scanning and treatment,
especially that due to respiration, may alter the location both of the tumor and of
adjacent normal structures relative to external or internal landmarks. Allowance

must be made for such potential changes, based on knowledge of how such movements can alter the contents of the treatment volume during actual therapy delivery. Currently available information relating to each of these four major problems will be discussed in detail below.

Registration of scan level to external or internal landmarks

Registration of level of transverse scan to external skin marks was accomplished in the above-cited studies by placing barium paste (JEM et al, 1977; Hobday et al, 1979) or radio-opaque catheters (Goitein et al, 1979) on skin reference marks during scanning.

The relationship of surface anatomic landmarks to vertebral level for determining scan level of cross-sectional images has been discussed by Kuhns et al (1978). Palpable external landmarks, including the tip of the xiphoid, the ends of the 11th rib, the umbilicus and the iliac crests, were studied in relation to corresponding vertebral segments as determined on anterior-posterior radiographs and abdominal scans in 50 patients undergoing intravenous urography. The location of the xiphoid ranged from the T_{10-11} interspace to the level of the 1st lumbar vertebral body; in 37 per cent of 35 patients the xiphoid was at the level of T_{11} or at the T_{11-12} interspace. The tip of the 11th rib was at the level of L_2, the L_{2-3} interspace or L_3 in 91 per cent of cases, and the umbilicus and the iliac crest at the L4, L4-5, or L5 level in 91 per cent and 98 per cent, respectively. It was concluded that these landmarks can be used only as a rough guide to approximate the level of abdominal organs for CT scanning, due to variability in organ level caused by body habitus and respiratory motion. Because the external landmarks studied were demonstrated to be relatively constantly related to vertebral segment, they were thought to be more reliable for localisation of the level of the vertebral bodies or of retroperitoneal structures which move relatively less with respiration than do the abdominal viscera.

Kreel (1977) has described a simple yet relatively accurate technique to relate scan level to vertebral level. Metal markers were placed over fixed bony points, such as the xiphoid, etc., and a radiograph was taken with a slit X-ray beam to minimise parallax. The level of each CT cut is then related to the radiograph and marked on that film, which becomes part of the patient's permanent radiographic record. A similar technique has been described by Dossetor et al (1979); a conventional radiograph is taken through a lead grid lattice with pinpoint holes separated by a distance equivalent to the thickness of the CT cuts, with aluminium markers placed on the skin at 5 cm intervals. The aluminum markers are left in place for the scan, produce no artifacts, and allow accurate registration of scan levels with vertebral levels on the AP radiograph.

Scan artifacts produced by external foreign objects in CT scanning fields, such as barium paste or other radio-opaque skin markers, can hinder accurate tissue boundary localisation and also interfere with quantitative use of CT numbers for tissue heterogeneity corrections in radiotherapy treatment planning. The Temple CT level indicator, described by Villafana et al, (1979), is said to allow relatively precise correlation between scan level and AP radiographs. It consists of a rectangular plexiglass plate with linear grooves 1 cm apart of lengths which vary in

1 cm increments. When placed under the patient at a previously marked level during scanning, the air filling the grooves is clearly seen on the scan, and the number of air spaces seen on any scan relates the level of that section to the external reference mark. A duplicate plate with copper wires filling the grooves is placed in the same position under the patient during simulation. When care was taken to exactly position the marking plate under the patient for both scanning and simulation, an overall accuracy of 5 mm was observed, with no artifacts being introduced.

Modification of scanners to allow a 'scout' film to be taken in the scanning position with appropriate markers projected on the film would simplify the task of registration of the scan section to the appropriate anatomic level of the patient. Availability of such films would greatly facilitate comparison of other studies such as arteriograms, etc. with the scan, and also be of significant value in radio-therapy treatment planning for comparison with simulator radiographs.

Effect of patient position on internal anatomy

The effect of *patient position* during the scan on organ and tumor location relative to fixed bony landmarks seen on the transverse image must be considered when using CT data in treatment planning. This can be of particular significance if either the tumor volume might move out of the treatment volume or if a dose-limiting organ might move into the treatment volume when patient position is other than that which is obtained during scanning. The potential utility of the scan for determining kidney position for shielding purposes during radiotherapy has been alluded to by Sagel et al (1977). Hobday and associates (1979) found that renal position on the scan differed from that determined with conventional techniques in 5 of 9 patients studied. Neither author specifically mentioned the possibility of renal position changes due to different patient position for treatment than had been used for scanning although the latter stressed the importance of performing the scan used for treatment planning in the treatment position. Haaga (1976) has observed organ shifts on scans performed in the supine and the right decubitus position. A pancreatic tumor could be seen more clearly in the latter position due to anterior and inferior shifts of the stomach, duodenum and liver away from the tumor; in the supine scan, those organs lay directly on the pancreas. In the decubitus scan, the left kidney moved anteromedially, and more of the right kidney was visualised, relative to renal position seen on the supine scan.

Lee et al (1979) have studied patients with gastric malignancies in the supine, prone, and decubitus positions, and found that the shift in the stomach and its contents with positional change allowed evaluation of the thickness of the anterior and posterior walls, which were outlined alternately by air and contrast material in the different positions.

Changes in organ and possibly tumor mass location may also occur after surgery, and care must be taken in using preoperative scans for treatment planning, especially if extensive extirpative surgery has been performed. Bernardino et al (1979) have studied anatomical changes occuring after nephrectomy with CT, observing that the post-nephrectomy renal fossa normally contains only bowel. Alter et al (1979) have also studied post-nephrectomy patients with CT, and state that the right renal fossa may be occupied by liver, colon, and the junction of the

2nd and 3rd portions of the duodenum. Following left nephrectomy, multiple loops of small bowel may occupy the left renal fossa, with the spleen and descending colon being located more postero-medially than their usual location. The tail of the pancreas was also observed to occupy the medial left renal bed, while after splenectomy and nephrectomy, the descending colon was seen there.

Shift in renal position between the supine and the prone position also occurs, as demonstrated by comparing a prone abdominal scan obtained for planning purposes in a cervical cancer patient with a follow-up scan done in the supine position. Prone scan sections at the levels of the first and second lumbar vertebral bodies are shown in Figures 14.1A and B, and supine scans are shown in Figures 14.1C and D. Note the loss of contrast from the lymphangiographically opacified

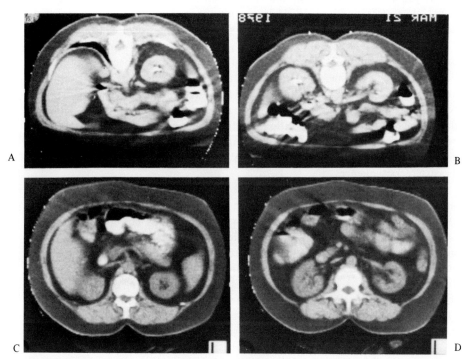

Fig. 14.1A & 1B (upper left and right). Prone scan at level of L₁ (left) and L₂ (right) of patient with cervix cancer metastatic to para aortic nodes.
Fig. 14.1C & 1D. Supine scan at same levels. Both scans done after oral and i.v. contrast. Note anteromedial displacement of kidneys in prone scans.

nodes which has occurred in the 20 months between the scans. The left kidney is seen on both upper and lower scans and the right only on the lower scan. The left kidney on both levels and the right on the lower level scan are more anteromedially located on the prone scan (Fig. 14.1A and B) relative to their position on the supine scan (Fig. 14.1C and D). The degree of displacement is modest, being 19, 14 and 16 mm in the antero-posterior direction and 9, 3 and 9 mm in the transverse direction for the left kidney at both levels and the right kidney at the lower level, respectively. The anterior-posterior and transverse diameters of the kidneys at these levels ranged from 5.0 to 6.6 cm. Thus, the observed kidney shift from the prone to the supine position approximates 1/3 (27-37 per cent) of the AP renal diameter and 10 per cent (5-15 per cent) of the transverse diameter at these levels. These shifts have obvious significance in terms of planning renal shielding based on renal position taken from the scan: with anterior and posterior para-aortic portals, the medial portion of the kidney might be completely excluded from the treatment field in the supine position and included in the prone position. The anterior renal margin might be excluded from lateral portals directed at the pancreatic area in the supine position, and included to a significant degree if treatment were to be given with the patient prone. Similarly, more posteriorly placed lateral portals directed at the para-aortic area would cover less than half of the kidney area with the patient supine, and include almost the entire organ if the patient were treated in the prone position. Similar renal shifts occur, as noted above (Haaga et al, 1976) in moving the patient from the supine to the decubitus position, and may also occur in going from the recumbent to the upright position. Further studies in this regard are planned when an EMI prototype scanner capable of scanning in both vertical and horizontal modes becomes available in the Radiation Medicine Department at the Massachusetts General Hospital in mid-1980. The quantitative nature of the measurements in this single patient can be questioned, since the scans were separated by a 20 month interval. However, the message is clear: kidney position does vary between the prone and the supine position, and renal localisation for shielding purposes must be done in the position in which treatment will be delivered or significant errors can occur, with potentially disastrous consequences.

Similar shifts of liver, small bowel, stomach, and the mobile portions of the large intestine, as well as the pancreas, occur with positional change as documented by Gunderson (1979). Figure 14.2A shows a prone small bowel film in a caecal carcinoma patient following right ileo-colectomy. The barium-filled small bowel and colon are relatively evenly distributed over the entire abdomen, and significant bowel is seen lateral to the sacro-iliac joint in the tumor bed overlying the right iliac fossa. However, when the patient is placed in the left lateral decubitus position (Fig. 14.2B), almost all the visualised bowel is medial to the S-I joint. Tumor bed irradiation given with AP and PA portals in that position would irradiate a significantly smaller volume of both small and large intestine than would have been treated with the same technique and portals with the patient prone. Significant displacement of bowel out of the target volume could be achieved by treating in the decubitus position when the target volume includes the lateral abdominal gutters, the iliac fossa, or the iliac bone itself. The degree of bowel displacement could be quantified by scanning the patient after administration of oral contrast in both the supine or prone position and in the appropriate decubitus position. Patients can be positioned for scanning and treatment with a simple decubitus board, as described and illustrated by Gunderson (1979).

Effects of involuntary patient motion on use of CT scan in treatment planning

Involuntary patient motion, especially respiration and peristalsis, degraded the diagnostic image in scans done with 1st generation scanners with relatively long scan times. However, these problems have been largely eliminated for imaging

A   B

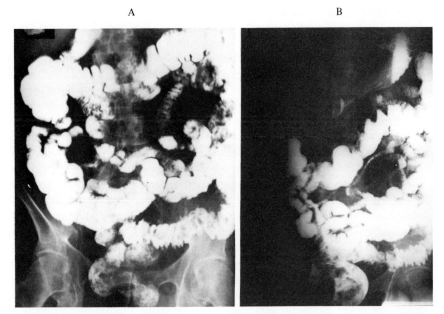

Fig. 14.2A & B Small bowel series in prone position (left) and left lateral decubitus position (right). Note displacement of bowel to left in decubitus position.

purposes by use of i.v. glucagon to inhibit peristalsis, and development of faster scanners which can complete a scan section during a single suspended respiration by the patient. Sagel et al (1977) have reported that 91 per cent of 131 patients with renal masses were able to suspend respiration for at least the 18 seconds required to complete a single scan. However, few therapy units can complete treatment in less than 18 seconds, and hence abdominal organ mobility with respiration must be considered in planning abdominal radiotherapy.

Kuhns et al (1979) have studied variation in renal and diaphragmatic position with repeated suspension of respiration in 32 patients undergoing intravenous urography. The position of the superior pole of the kidney on 1, 2 and 3 minute films in the same patient had mean variations ranging from 4.9 to 7.7 mm despite the patient being given the same specific breathing instructions for each film. The apex of the diaphragm was seen on each film in 12 patients: mean variation in diaphragm position was 8.0 mm. These data were cited to emphasize the difficulty of scanning an identical level on subsequent scans, due to internal organ mobility with respiration, and to demonstrate that internal anatomy cannot be voluntarily reproduced even by co-operative patients.

Haaga and associates (1977) have noted that increased pressure from the weight of the abdominal viscera in the right lateral decubitus position decreased right diaphragmatic excursion and aided visualisation of the pancreas on abdominal scans. Kivisarri et al (1979) observed that the pancreas moved with respiration as much as two vertebral segments, and cited this great mobility as an impediment to re-scanning an identical abdominal section. The stomach, duodenum, kidney and liver probably move as much as the pancreas, although CT data in this regard are lacking.

The effect of respiration on treatment planning was studied by Hobday and associates (1979) who detected contour change in 6 of 19 (32 per cent) abdominal patients, with a significant change in plan occuring in 2 of the 19 (10.5 per cent). In those 2, respiration caused anterior displacement of the isocenter which moved the treatment volume off the tumor during treatment. No significant changes due to respiration were noted in 65 pelvic or 30 thoracic patients studied. Scans were performed with suspended respiration for diagnostic purposes, and the area of interest re-scanned during quiet respiration. Scan sections were subsequently superimposed to detect changes in body contour or internal anatomy due to breathing conditions likely to be existing during treatment. It was explicitely stated that no transverse motion of either internal organs or of the tumor was detected during quiet breathing. No axial organ or tumor movement was described.

The implications of respiratory motion of abdominal organs for treatment planning are significant. Accurate saggital and coronal reconstructions would be extremely valuable in treatment planning since they would allow three dimensional comprehension of tumor extent in a format similar to the AP and lateral radiographs usually obtained from treatment simulators. However, Foley and associates (1979) have suggested that resolution of saggital and coronal reconstructions is limited by scan thickness and by anatomic overlap of contiguous scan sections due to patient respiration. To avoid errors in reconstructions due to changes in internal anatomy with time because of the respiratory excursion of mobile abdominal organs during sequential abdominal scans, Kuhns et al (1979) have suggested that multiple scans at contiguous levels during a single suspension of respiration may be required to obtain accurate density data for reconstruction in other planes.

The therapist must realise that tumors or organs seen on any given transverse section may not be there, relative to fixed vertebral landmarks or to skin marks, during the entire length of the treatment and that other tissues may replace those seen on any given section due to respiratory motion of mobile abdominal organs. If the tumor involves a mobile organ, such as the pancreas, stomach or kidney, the treatment volume must be large enough to include the tumor in all phases of respiration, unless techniques can be devised to gait treatment to the respiratory cycle. If a high dose rate (500 rads/minute) therapy unit is available, co-operative patients can be treated in a particular phase of respiration, although the variation in diaphragmatic and renal position in 'co-operative patients' cited above suggests that significant margins are still required when tumors involving mobile abdominal organs are irradiated. Allowance should also be made for kidney mobility with respiration when renal blocks are made for shielding purposes.

Movement of mobile tumors or organs in the anterior-posterior direction with respiration has not been evaluated, either with CT or with conventional techniques. Further studies are urgently needed to confirm that the rate of 'significant' change in treatment plans with respiration is no greater than the 10 per cent change found by Hobday et al (1979) due to anterior abdominal wall skin excursion with respiration.

Quantification of tissue inhomogeneities for abdominal treatment planning

Tissue inhomogeneities may produce significant variations in dose distribution, especially if electrons or charged particles are employed. Inhomogeneities of interest in abdominal treatment planning include vertebral bone, subcutaneous, retroperitoneal and intraperitoneal fat, and air cavities in bowel or external to the patient, as illustrated in Figures 14.1A-D. For supervoltage photon beams, the presence of fat or bone in the field produces an insignificant change in dose distribution, and can hence be ignored. The presence of air in bowel could produce significant alterations in dose distribution. However, patients undergoing daily fractionated radiotherapy would probably have varying amounts of air in the bowel, occupying different positions from day to day. Transmission measurements during fractionated pelvic or abdominal irradiation could quantitate dose variations due to different amounts of air in the bowel from day to day as suggested by Dische & Zanelli (1976). However, such measurements do not reveal if the offending air is in the entrance or the exit dose region, relative to the target volume. Hence they would be of limited value for use on a day-to-day basis to compensate for varying amounts of air in the gut which would affect dose distribution within the target volume during fractionated radiotherapy. A satisfactory way of dealing with this problem would be to scan the treatment volume immediately prior to treatment, with appropriate compensation being made on a day-to-day basis. A worthwhile study in a radiotherapy department with a dedicated scanner would be to scan the same section through the treatment volume daily to determine the variation of air in the gut on a day-to-day basis; the effect of diet, drugs and other factors on gut air could also be assessed in such a study.

Alterations in external contour which might be missed with a conventionally obtained contour can be detected on the scan; such a situation is illustrated in Figures 14.1C and D, where the posterior air gap between the table top and the skin surface approximates 2 cm. If uncompensated, the air gap would introduce an overdose to the midplane of the patient's abdomen created with equally weighted anterior and posterior portals directed to the pancreas or para-aortic area of 5 per cent, 3 per cent and 1.5 per cent with Co^{60}, 10 MV and 25 MV X-rays, respectively.

Comparative treatment planning

Modern radiotherapy departments typically have the potential to employ various modalities with isocentric treatment units which can direct the beam to the volume of interest from any desired direction. At the Massachusetts General Hospital, there are available isocentrically configured units delivering Cobalt-60 gamma rays and 10 and 25 MV photons, as well as nine electron beams ranging in energy from 4MeV to 35 MeV. A fixed horizontal 160 MeV proton beam is also available. Computerised treatment planning capability exists or is being developed to combine any of these beams to treat a specific volume of interest. Optimised plans for alternate treatments with various modalities can be developed; frequently it is not obvious which plan is superior, since all can deliver the desired dose to the target volume and keep the dose to a specific critical organ, such as the kidney or spinal cord, to below tolerance levels. A simple calculation of integral dose on each plan could form the basis for comparison of plans, but the plan with the lowest integral dose might still approach or exceed the tolerance of a dose-limiting normal structure. Determination of differential normal tissue doses for each plan would allow quantitative comparison of plans which all treat the tumor volume adequately. Transverse CT sections display the tumor and its relationship to normal dose-limiting organs. The tumor, the target volume and the location of sensitive normal structures can all be identified on the scan and transferred directly or indirectly to the treatment planning computer. Plans could be generated to treat the tumor volume to the desired dose, and plots made of dose distribution to normal structures with each plan. The plan which gives the lowest dose to the normal structures would then be quantitatively superior to other plans and could be chosen for use. An alternative approach would be to specify maximum allowed dose for a specific structure, e.g., the spinal cord, and determine what dose the target volume and other normal tissues would receive with alternate plans. An example of the latter technique will be discussed below.

The target volume and sensitive normal structures, including spinal cord, kidneys, and bowel on a patient with pancreatic cancer have been traced from an enlarged projection of a CT section at the L-2 level in a patient with pancreatic cancer, and are shown in Figure 14.3. This contour was then input into the PC 12

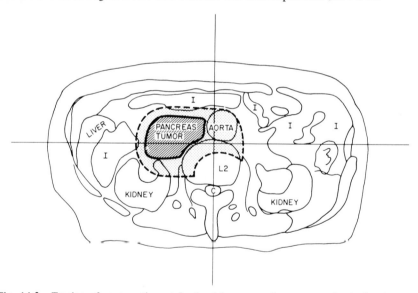

Fig. 14.3 Tracing of scan section at L_2 level in pancreatic cancer patient, showing tumor (cross hatched with solid border) and target volume (stippled with broken border) as well as normal structures seen at this level. C is spinal cord, I is intestine and L_2 is second lumbar vertebral body.

treatment planning computer, and optimised 2-field (anterior and posterior, equally weighted portals) and 4-field (anterior, posterior, right and left lateral, weighted 2:2:1:1, respectively) treatment plans were generated with Co^{60} gamma rays and 25 MV X-rays. Cord tolerance of 5000 rads was taken as the limiting factor, and the doses to the target volume to the kidneys and to the bowel were determined with that constraint. Doses to these areas with the 4 plans studied are shown in Table 14.5. Tolerance of the right kidney, defined as more than 2000 rads to over 50 per

Table 14.5 Comparative dosimetry to pancreatic tumor volume

Technique	Dose to specified regions when spinal cord dose 5000 rads				
	Target volume rads	% kidney right	2000 rads left	% bowel 5000	4000
2-field* Co-60	4650	100	0	0	20
25-X	4900	95	5	0	25
4-field** Co-60	5450	100	20	15	30
25-X	6000	98	25	20	30

*Equally weighted anterior and posterior portals.
**Anterior, posterior, right and left lateral portals with relative weighting of 2:2:1:1

cent of the organ, is exceeded with all plans when cord tolerance is the dose limiting factor, but none of the plans exceeds the specified tolerance of the left kidney. A small percentage of the bowel exceeds the defined tolerance level of 5000 rads with each of the 4-field plans. A significantly higher dose can be given to the target volume with the 4-field 25 MV X-ray plan than with any of the other plans, while not exceeding defined tolerance levels of the spinal cord and of the left kidney. The therapist could then make a clinical judgement based on clinical experience, bowel mobility studies, patient tolerance and other factors, whether to push the dose to the 6000 rad level or to stop at a lower dose which carries with it a lesser probability of disease sterilisation within the irradiated volume, but also a lesser risk of small bowel injury. Simple field arrangements were chosen to illustrate the technique. Other more sophisticated techniques with varied angulations, weightings, beam modifiers, etc. could be chosen, which might allow a greater dose to be delivered to the target volume while not exceeding normal tissue tolerance as defined. For maximum safety, planning at other levels should also be done, since tolerance to a critical structure or structures might be exceeded at other levels throughout the treated volume although specified tolerance levels were not exceeded on the section initially studied. Such an exercise would be prohibitively costly if done by manual techniques, but treatment planning programs could be developed to direct the computer to carry out such computations automatically, expressing results as the percentage of each critical organ which receives a dose greater than the maximum defined tolerance dose for that organ when the tumor volume receives a particular dose, or when the dose to one critical structure is taken as the primary constraint, as has been shown in the example cited.

Summary and conclusions

The radiotherapy community has begun to appreciate the significant contribution which CT can make to planning abdominal radiotherapy, and is also beginning to appreciate the pitfalls and limitations of the technique. Specific attention must now be focused on problems relating to patient registration with the scanner and

132

with simulator radiographs, patient position during scanning and treatment, and effects of involuntary patient motion, especially breathing on organ and tumor location. Further efforts are also needed to quantitate the effects of patient positional changes and immobilisation errors and motion during treatment on treatment planning and execution, and to study effects of inhomogeneities, especially gut air on abdominal dose distribution. Radiotherapy with CT assistance has the potential to impact significantly on morbidity and mortality associated with abdominal malignancies. Radiotherapists, radiodiagnosticians, radiation physicists, and oncologists must meet the challenge of realising that potential for the benefit of the cancer patients entrusted to their care.

References

Alter A J, Uehling D T, Zwiebel W J 1979 Computed tomography of the retroperitoneum following nephrectomy. Radiology 133: 663-668

Bernardino M E, deSantos L A, Johnson D E, Bracken R B 1979 Computed tomography in the evaluation of post-nephrectomy patients. Radiology 130: 183-187

Dische S, Zanelli J D 1976 Bowel gas — a cause of elevated dose in radiotherapy. British Journal of Radiology 30: 543-549

Dossetor R S, Veiga-Pires J A, Kaiser M 1979 Localisation of scanning level in computed tomography of the spine. Journal of Computer Assisted Tomography 3 (2): 284-285

Ferrucci J T Jr, Wittenberg J 1978 CT biopsy of abdominal tumors: aids for lesion localisation. Radiology 129: 739-744

Foley W D, Lawson T L, Quiroz F 1979 Sagittal and coronal image reconstruction: application in pancreatic computed tomography. Journal of Computer Assisted Tomography 3 (6): 717-721

Goitein M, Wittenberg J, Mendiondo M, Doucette J, Freidberg C, Ferrucci J, Gunderson L, Linggood R, Shipley W U, Fineberg H V 1979 The value of CT scanning in radiation therapy treatment planning: a prospective study. International Journal Radiation Oncology, Biology, Physics 5: 1787-1798

Gunderson L 1979 Radiation Oncology. In: Margulis A R, Burhenne H J (ed) Alimentary tract radiology. Abdominal imaging volume 3. Mosby, St Louis, ch 44, 600-619

Haaga J R, Alfidi R J, Zelch M G, Meany T F, Boller M, Gonzalez L, Jelden G L 1976 Computed tomography of the pancreas. Radiology 120: 589-595

Hobday P, Hodson N J, Husband J, Parker R P, Macdonald J S 1979 Computed tomography applied to radiotherapy treatment planning: techniques and results. Radiology 133: 477-482

Kivisaari L, Kormano M, Rantakokko V 1979 Contrast enhancement of the pancreas in computed tomography. Journal of Computer Assisted Tomography 3 (6): 722-726

Kreel L 1977 Computerised tomography using the EMI general purpose scanner. British Journal of Radiology 50: 2-14

Kuhns L R, Borlaza G S, Seigel R, Thornbury J R 1978 External anatomic landmarks of the abdomen related to vertebral segments: applications in cross-sectional imaging. American Journal of Roentgenology 131: 115-117

Kuhns L R, Thornbury J, Seigel R 1979 Variation of position of the kidneys and diaphragm in patients undergoing repeated suspension of respiration. Journal of Computer Assisted Tomography 3 (5): 620-621

Lee J K T, Levitt R G, Stanley R J, Sagel S S 1978 Utility of body computed tomography in the clinical follow-up of abdominal masses. Journal of Computer Assisted Tomography 2: 607-611

Lee K R, Levine E, Moffat R E, Bigongiari L R, Hermreck A S 1979 Computed tomographic staging of malignant gastric neoplasms. Radiology 133: 151-155

Munzenrider J E, Pilepich M, Rene-Ferrero J B, Tchakarova I, Carter B L 1977 Use of body scanner in radiotherapy treatment planning. Cancer 40: 170-179

Pilepich M, Rene J B, Munzenrider J E, Carter B L 1978 Contribution of computed tomography to the treatment of lymphomas. American Journal of Roentgenology 131: 670-673

Sagel S S, Stanley R J, Levitt R G, Geisse G 1977 Computed tomography of the kidney. Radiology 124: 359-370

Villafana T, Lee S H, Vider M, Wu R K 1979 Device for correlating CT and radiation therapy portal images. American Journal of Roentgenology 133: 1191-1193

Wittenberg J, Ferrucci J T Jr 1978 Computed body tomography. Gastroenterology 74: 287-293

15. The practical implementation of CT for radiotherapy treatment planning

J. R. CUNNINGHAM and J. VAN DYK

Introduction

It is stated in ICRU Report 24 (ICRU, 1976) that $\pm$ 5 per cent is a reasonable degree of accuracy to strive for in the delivery of the prescribed dose in radiotherapy. At least five steps are involved in this process; the calibration of the dosimeter, its use in the field in a reference phantom for machine calibrations, dose calculation in a 'water equivalent' patient, allowance for tissue inhomogeneity and actual delivery of the dose. A limit of $\pm$ 5 per cent on the sum of all of these steps is very demanding.

Until the advent of the CT scanner the required delineation of anatomical structures was just not available. With the advent of the CT scanner this was suddenly no longer true and the onus is cleanly on physics to develop a method of dose calculation that will meet the required degree of accuracy.

Physical problems

In Figure 15.1 we look at some of the problems from a physical point of view. A point, P, in a heterogeneous phantom receives primary radiation that comes directly along path d. The dose from this component depends on all of the material traversed by this path. Point P also receives radiation that is scattered once by a volume labelled dV and therefore depends on the material along paths a and b, on the scattering angle θ as well as the material making up dV. In addition there will be multiple scattered radiation that involves all other possible paths. The problem, in short, is a three dimensional one and is very complicated because the dose at P depends on all of the material irradiated and its location relative to point P. Figure 15.2 illustrates an attempt to try to assess the relative importance of each of these three components; primary, once scattered and multiple scattered radiation. The data is for a point at a depth of 10 cm in a water phantom irradiated by a series of beams (of increasing radius) from a cobalt unit. The ordinate is the percentage of the total dose that is due to each of the components. The primary and once scattered component can be calculated directly, the multiple scatter component is inferred by comparing the results of these calculations to measured (tissue-air ratio) data. The importance of scattered radiation can be seen to increase rapidly with field size and for a beam radius of 11 cm (approximately a 20x20 beam), accounts for over 1/3 of the total dose. Multiple scattered radiation accounts for over 20 per cent of the total.

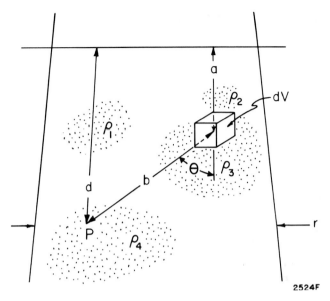

Fig. 15.1 Point P is in a homogeneous phantom. It receives radiation that comes to it directly and after being scattered from all other locations that are irradiated such as dV.

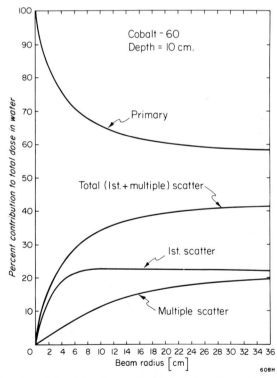

Fig. 15.2 Graphs showing relative importance of primary and scatter components to absorbed dose at a point 10 cm deep in radiation beams from a cobalt unit.

136

The use of Monte Carlo methods is being explored, for example by Webb & Parker (1978) and the results are useful for clarifying ideas but this approach is not practical for routine patient calculations with the present state of computer technology. A compromise solution, called the 'equivalent tissue-air ratio method' has been proposed by Sontag & Cunningham (1978) which has proven to be practical yet appears to involve little sacrifice in accuracy and furthermore lends itself easily to the direct use of the information provided by the CT scanner.

The equivalent tissue-air ratio method

1. Principles

The essence of this method is the idea, put forth by O'Connor (1957), that such quantities as tissue-air ratios could be obtained for phantoms made of non water equivalent material by scaling depth and field size by the density of the material. The implication of this is illustrated in Figure 15.3, where two phantoms whose densities differ by a factor two are compared. A practical procedure is accordingly set up to determine the equivalent electron density of a patient. A two step procedure is adopted. First the doses are calculated assuming a water equivalent

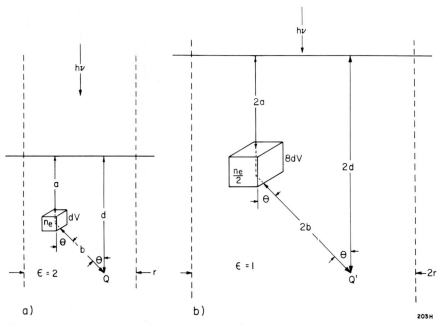

a)   b)   203H

Fig. 15.3 Diagram illustrating the scaling of tissue-air ratios for phantoms of different densities. Point Q, in a phantom of relative electron density 2 receives the same radiation dose as does point Q' in a phantom of relative electron density 1. All linear dimensions are scaled by the ratio of the densities and both doses are relative to the dose in air at the same points.

patient. As a second step a correction factor is obtained for each point which is made up of a ratio of two tissue-air ratios:

$$C = \frac{T(d', \hat{r})}{T(d,r)} \qquad \text{(equation 1)}$$

where d is the depth and r is the (equivalent) field radius and D and r are the scaled values of these two quantities.

The procedure for determining the scaled depth and field size is easy in principle but in its practical implementation a number of approximations must be made. For primary radiation the scaling would be given by:

$$d = d \cdot \sum_{j=1}^{n} \epsilon_j \qquad \text{(equation 2)}$$

where ϵ_j are the relative electron densities along path d. For scattered radiation the whole of the irradiated volume must be considered and an average density could be defined as follows:

$$\hat{\rho} = \frac{\sum_i \sum_j \sum_k w_{ijk} \; \epsilon_{ijk}}{\sum_i \sum_j \sum_k w_{ijk}} \qquad \text{(equation 3)}$$

where the ϵ_{ijk} are the relative electron densities (CT pixels converted to electron densities) of the tissues and the w_{ijk} are weighting factors which are intended to express the relative importance of each of the ijk volume elements in contributing scattered radiation to the point of calculation.

There is no 'correct' set of weighting factors. They would in principle be different for each point of calculation, as well as for each configuration of tissues. An experiment by Andrew et al (1979) gives an indication of the expected form of them. Their results are shown in Figure 15.4. An ionisation chamber was positioned as indicated in a water phantom and rings of polystyrene foam of various radii were placed, alternately, at various depths. The foam is of very low density and represented the replacement of water by volumes of air. The readings, with and without the foam in place were noted and 'iso-effect' lines were drawn. They express the change in scattered radiation reaching the dosimeter that is caused by replacing a unit volume (1 cm^3) of water by air.

The results are somewhat surprising. They show, for example, that at some locations, the result of replacing water by air is an increase in scatter, while at others there is a decrease. The weighting factors required for equation 3 would have a form similar to the lines in this diagram.

2. Calculations

Direct evaluation of the summation in equation 3 would involve an integration over the entire irradiated volume for each point of calculation. Although this would be much shorter than a Monte Carlo calculation it was still considered impractical at the present time so a compromise procedure which is indicated in Figure 15.5 was adopted. On the left is depicted 6 CT slices. Dose calculations are to be made in the shaded one. The first step is to reduce, or coalesce, all of the density information of the six slices into one 'effective' slice as shown on the right. A method of doing this is discussed by Sontag & Cunningham (1978) and will not

138

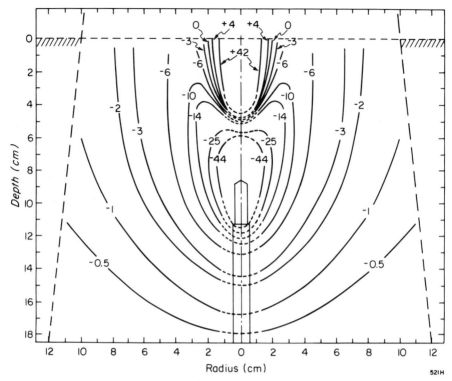

Fig. 15.4 Diagram of 'iso-effect curves' for scattered radiation. Each curve links regions in a water phantom where the introduction of a styrofoam inhomogeneity has an equal effect on the dose as measured at the ionisation chamber. The numbers, when divided by 1000, give the percentage change in total dose per cm^3 of water displaced by styrofoam.

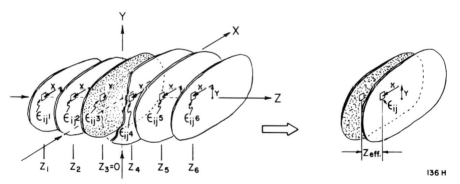

Fig. 15.5 Schematic diagram illustrating the steps taken in evaluating the 'effective density' for scattered radiation. Six CT slices are irradiated from above. The densities in all six slices are 'coalesced' to form a weighted average, or effective slice shown on the right. It is then considered to be at an effective distance, Zeff, from the plane of calculation which is shown dotted. As a final step a weighted average overall density is obtained for each point of calculation.

be repeated here. This 'coalescing' is performed only once for the whole (shaded) plane and by this means the volume integration is reduced to an integration over a plane. This makes the procedure practical both with respect to time and space in the computer. The correction factor of equation 1 is then evaluated for each point and the corrected dose distribution is obtained.

Implementation

1. Procedures

To employ CT for radiation therapy planning we have modified a computerised treatment planning system (TP-11 of Atomic Energy of Canada, Ltd) to interface with a CT scanner (Picker X-ray Corporation, model Synerview-600), as shown in Figure 15.6. The scanner is operated jointly by the radiotherapy and diagnostic radiology departments. A patient being scanned for radiotherapy purposes is

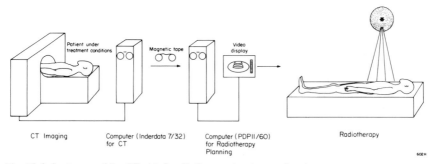

Fig. 15.6 System used for CT-aided radiotherapy treatment planning.

positioned by radiotherapy staff (including technical staff) on the scanner couch in the same position they will have when they are treated. They breathe normally during a 20 second or so CT scan to provide average locations and densities of tissues (Battista, 1979). The CT data are then transferred, via magnetic tape to the treatment planning computer, where the 'CT numbers' are converted to electron densities for purposes of dose calculation. The images taken in planes in which dose calculations are to be made may be used to determine external contour outlines of the patient and may be displayed to show tissues relative to treatment fields and corresponding radiation dose distributions. Slice images in the plane of dose calculation and planes on either side of it (spanning the volume irradiated) are used to make allowance for the effect of tissue inhomogeneities as described. The patient is treated on a radiotherapy unit in the same position and following it the patient may again be examined by CT to follow the response of the diseased and healthy tissues.

2. Comparison: conventional versus CT-aided procedures

The CT-aided treatment planning system considered here has been under development for several years and has been in routine clinical use since August 1978.

140

Figure 15.7 shows a block diagram comparing conventional to CT-aided treatment planning procedures. For both techniques a patient is referred for treatment with

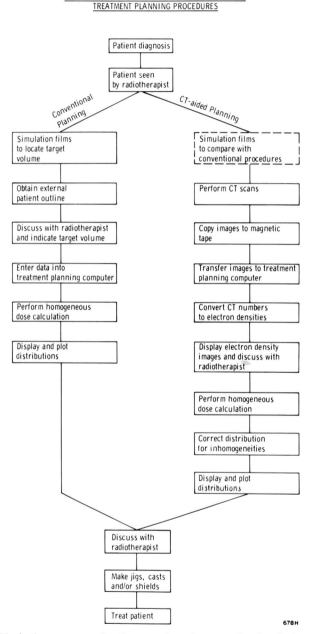

Fig. 15.7 Block diagram comparing the procedures in conventional radiotherapy planning to CT-aided planning.

an established diagnosis. The radiation oncologist then proposes a treatment procedure. In the conventional approach, radiographs are obtained from a therapy simulator and an external outline of the patient is determined. The radiation oncologist delineates the target volume and the location of critical structures with respect to this outline. These data are then entered into a treatment planning computer for selection of appropriate radiation beams. One or more dose distributions are calculated assuming the tissues are of water-like density and presented to the radiation oncologist for approval. Following discussions with the physics and technical staff, preparations are made to initiate the treatment.

CT aided planning is more complex. Again, the patient may be referred to the simulator for examination although in many instances the CT scanner replaces the simulator. The patient is placed on the CT scanner couch in the exact position that will be used for treatment and CT scans of the proposed irradiation volume are performed. For this a flat insert for the concave scanner couch has been provided. Reference markers are placed on the patient using thin solder wire, 0.1 cm in diameter and 0.5 cm long. These markers can be readily observed on the CT images, yet are small enough to avoid the production of serious image artifacts. Contrast media are also used to aid in delineating structures when necessary; however, high concentrations must be avoided, since this would introduce errors into the dosage computations.

The resultant CT images are stored on magnetic tape and are transferred to the treatment planning computer where the CT numbers are converted to electron densities using the approach suggested by Battista et al (1980). The images can be displayed on the treatment planning computer for the radiotherapist to define the target and critical volumes. This latter procedure implies a meeting between clinical, physics and technical staff at the computer and has the side benefit of encouraging interaction between them.

Using electron densities directly, an external patient contour is calculated and a dose distribution is determined first assuming internal tissues to be of water-like density. This dose distribution forms the link with past clinical experience but is subsequently corrected for the actual tissue densities utilising the equivalent tissue-air ratio method proposed by Sontag & Cunningham (1978). This calculation uses the CT data of all of the slices covering the entire irradiated volume, hence changes in external contours and internal anatomical structures are accounted for. Any of the images may be displayed or obtained full size on an electrostatic printer plotter for examination. The final distribution, with the isodose curves superimposed on the CT image, is discussed with the radiation oncologist and preparations are made for implementing the treatment as prescribed.

Summary of practical experience

At the present time in our clinic, CT-aided radiotherapy planning requires about twice as much time as conventional procedures. In due course, with more sophisticated hardware and software this time differential will be reduced. As part of a general evaluation procedure we have applied CT scanning to a number of sites with the intent of determining the factors most likely to affect tissue-localisation and the behaviour of dose distributions. Table 15.1 lists 174 patients that were scanned between August 1978 to September 1979. In this same time interval, over 2500 patients were scanned during the diagnostic time period. Since our hospital is a specialised institution dealing with malignant diseases, many of the diagnostic studies may also have had some effect on the treatment technique although the impact of this is difficult to assess. As shown in this table 43 per cent of the 174 patients were scanned for tissue localisation to determine position of radiation fields. In the remaining 57 per cent, the scan data was used to determine dose distributions. CT scans of the thorax region were employed more frequently for computing dose distributions than any other site (35 per cent of the patients studied). This is as expected since the effects of tissue inhomogeneities are much greater in the thorax than other sites. Since these patients were not placed in a prospective study, it is difficult to determine exactly how many of them had changes in their treatment technique as a result of information provided by the scans. However, as a first approximation, we estimate that over 50 per cent of these patients had a change in prescribed dose or in the treatment procedure as a result of the additional information provided by CT.

Table 15.1 CT-aided radiotherapy planning (August 17, 1978 to September 10, 1979)

Site	Number of patients	Purpose	
		Tissue localisation or densitometry(%)	Dose computation (%)
Head	19	7	2
Thorax	73	6	35
Abdomen	30	13	5
Pelvis	41	10	13
Other	11	7	2
Totals	174	43	57

Special studies

1. Half body irradiation and radiation pneumonitis

The use of half body irradiation was pioneered at our institute by Rider & Fitzpatrick (1976). Because this technique was found to provide an excellent means of palliation for disseminated malignant disease, it is now being used more often as an adjunct to other therapeutic procedures or even as a form of primary treatment. However, one of the major concerns of upper half body irradiation is lung toxicity. Results reported by Fryer et al (1979) indicated an incidence of radiation pneumonitis of 29 per cent for 800 rad and of 84 per cent for 1000 rad tissue dose to the upper half body given by cobalt-60 radiation in a single fraction. Originally, these doses were administered assuming the patient consisted of waterlike tissues without corrections for lung inhomogeneities. In order to limit the doses to lung to non toxic levels, the factors affecting the dose to lung must be clearly understood.

We have studied a group of 23 patients using our CT-aided treatment planning system. External patient contours, the geometry of the internal structures and the relative electron density of these structures were derived from the CT scans. Two dose distributions were determined for each patient. The first distribution was calculated assuming the patient is composed of unit density tissues. The second distribution included corrections to account for the actual electron densities throughout the irradiated volume. A pair of typical distributions are illustrated in Figure 15.8. For the purposes of determining maximum dose correction factors as well as average electron densities, measurements were made along the dashed vertical lines illustrated in Figure 15.8. The most pertinent results obtained from this group of patients are summarised in Table 15.2.

Table 15.2 Summary of measured parameters for 38 normal lungs

	Average	Minimum	Maximum
Total patient thickness	21.9	17.2	25.8
Total lung thickness	14.2	8.3	19.6
Average electron density for lung	0.244	0.169	0.343
Maximum dose correction factor	1.164	1.099	1.244

In the process of analysing this data, other inhomogeneity calculation procedures were examined to test their accuracy for these extremely large cobalt-60 radiation fields. The linear attenuation method of a 3.5 per cent per cm correction and the 'effective attenuation method' as recommended by the ICRU (1976) yielded dose correction factors for the mid lung region that were approximately 12 per cent higher than those calculated by the equivalent TAR method. Conversely, the generalised Batho method of Sontag & Cunningham (1977) yielded dose correction factors that were 12 per cent lower. Because of these extremely large differences, measurements were performed in the lung region of the Alderson Rando phantom under the conditions of upper half body irradiation. For cobalt-60 radiation, the equivalent TAR method agreed with the measured data to within $\pm$ 2 per cent. Certainly, an awareness of the accuracy of the various inhomogeneity correction methods is essential when determining the dose to lung for large field radiotherapy.

To determine the dose to lung retrospectively for the group of patients in the study by Fryer et al (1978), the relationship between patient thickness and dose correction factor was studied. It was found that the calculated dose correction factors showed an extremely good linear correlation with the patient thickness. Indeed more than 80 per cent of the data points for normal lungs were within 1.5 per cent of the least squares fit straight line. As expected, points for abnormal lungs illustrate much greater discrepancies. Using this linear relationship, dose correction factors were then determined for the patients in Fryer's study. Patients with known abnormal lungs were excluded since their dose correction factors could be inaccurate. Figure 15.9 illustrates the incidence of radiation pneumonitis versus corrected dose to lung. For the sake of comparison Fryer's original data is shown by the dashed line. CT-aided planning has enabled the dose complication curve for radiation pneumonitis to be considered in terms of absolute dose to lung rather than the dose based on unit density tissues.

144

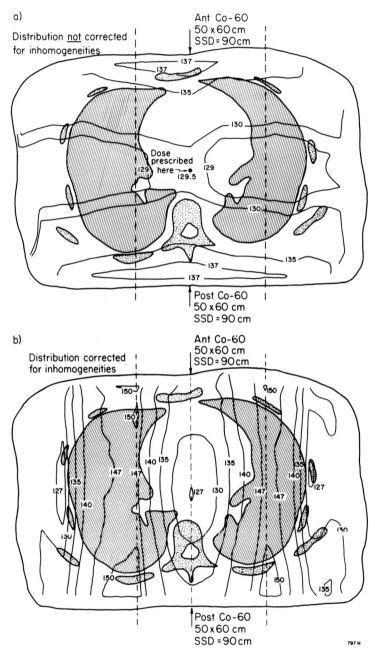

Fig. 15.8 Dose distributions for treatment of the upper half body. The lower diagram includes dose corrections for tissue inhomogeneities, the upper diagram does not. Density analysis have been carried out along the dashed lines, one of which is shown in Figure 15.10.

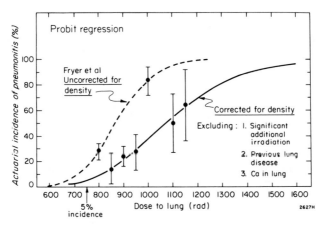

Fig. 15.9 Graph showing response versus dose curves for the incidence of radiation induced pneumonitis in healthy lungs. The correction for density was made retrospectively, based on a linear relationship obtained between patient thickness and dose correction factor.

2. Lung density analysis

As part of the radiation pneumonitis study, electron densities of lungs were analysed in some detail. Because CT provides a means of determining lung densities, in vivo, with an accuracy much greater than previously possible, a brief summary of our findings will be presented.

For each of the 23 patients of the upper half body irradiation project, electron density profiles were determined along the reference lines as illustrated by the dashed lines of Figure 15.8. An example, of such an electron density profile for a patient in the supine position is illustrated in Figure 15.10. The various anatomical regions are marked. Two regions of interest are the low and high density regions within the lung. When the same patient was rescanned in the prone position similar high and low density regions were again seen. The high density region however shifted from the anterior to the posterior side. This was likely to be due to gravitational blood pooling. From our measured data the following points are worth recording:

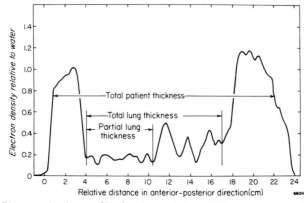

Fig. 15.10 Electron density profile showing variation of tissues along the left hand dashed line of Figure 15.8. The patient was lying prone and breathing normally during a 25 sec scan.

1. Lung thickness in the AP direction varies considerably from patient to patient. On average, the lung thickness is 0.64 of the total thickness. However, this approximation can lead to errors in lung thickness of 3 to 4 cm in some patients.

2. Local electron densities of lung averaged over at least a 2 cm path length can vary from 0.08 to greater than 0.40, differing from patient to patient as well as from one location to another within the same lung.

3. Abnormal lungs can display extreme variations from normal values. In one emphysematous patient, for example, the average density over the total lung length was 0.063.

4. Normal average lung densities were found to be age dependent. A plot of average lung density versus age for 68 normal lungs has indicated that average densities decrease from 0.36 at age 5 to 0.20 at age 80. This finding might be useful for dose calculations when CT is not available.

5. A group of 8 patients were analysed to determine the effects on lung densities of inspiration and expiration compared to normal breathing. With an average density of 0.289 for normal breathing, the average density for inspiration was 0.207 while the average density for expiration was 0.313. Certainly, fast scans under inspiration conditions yield large differences in the average density of lung. For treatment planning purposes, slow scans while the patient is breathing normally probably yields the best average electron density information even though the image may contain some additional motion artifacts.

References

Andrew J W, Van Dyk J, Johns H E 1979 Use of scattered radiation measurements in radiotherapy dose calculations based on computed tomography (CT) images. Proc. Soc. Photo-Optical Inst. Eng. 173: 342-347

Battista J J, Van Dyk J, Rider W D and Cunningham J R 1979 The application of computed tomographic (CT) imaging to radiotherapy planning. Proc. Soc. Photo-Optical Inst. Eng. 173: 348-353

Battista J J, Rider W D, Van Dyk J 1980 CT-aided radiotherapy planning. International Journal of Radiation, Oncology, Biology, Physics (in press)

Fitzpatrick P J, Rider W D 1976 Half body radiotherapy. International Journal of Radiation, Oncology, Biology, Physics 1: 197-207

Fryer C J H, Fitzpatrick P J, Rider W D, Poon P 1978 Radiation pneumonitis: experience following a large single dose of radiation. International Journal of Radiation, Oncology, Biology, Physics 4: 931-936

International Commission on Radiological Units and Measurements (ICRU) 1976 Report 24. Determination of absorbed dose in a patient irradiated by beams of X or gamma rays in radiotherapy procedures. Washington DC, USA

O'Connor J E 1957 The variation of scattered X-rays with density in an irradiated body. Physics in Medicine and Biology 1: 352-369

Sontag M R, Cunningham J R 1978 The equivalent tissue-air ratio method for making absorbed tomography for inhomogeneity corrections in photon beam dose calculations. Radiology 124: 143-149

Sontag M R, Cunningham J R 1977 Corrections to absorbed dose calculations for tissue inhomogeneities. Medical Physics 4: 431-436

Sontag M R, Cunningham J R 1978 The quivalent tissue-air ratio method for making absorbed dose calculations in a heterogeneous medium. Radiology 129: 787-794

Webb S, Parker R P 1978 A Monte Carlo study of the interaction of external beam x-radiation with inhomogeneous media. Physics in Medicine and Biology 23: 1043-1059

16. The use of CT data for inhomogeneity corrections in radiotherapy dose calculation

A. DUTREIX and A. BRIDIER

In order to ensure the required accuracy in dose delivery, accurate treatment planning is needed. This requires a knowledge of cross sectional anatomy for two main reasons: first, determination of the extent of the tumour and its localisation with respect to surrounding tissues and body outline; second, quantitative information on density distribution throughout the treated volume to enable corrections to be made for the attenuation of X-ray beams or the absorption of electron beams in different materials. We shall consider only this last aspect of treatment planning.

The relevant parameter for dose calculation in high energy X-ray therapy is the relative electron density ρ_{eh} of the tissues h under consideration, if one assumes that interaction of photons takes place primarily by the Compton process. Dose distribution in the presence of medium h is usually calculated by applying correction factors CF to the dose distribution calculated in water. In a similar way in high energy electron therapy the relevant parameter is the relative electron density ρ_{eh} since the slowing-down of electrons is governed by the number of electrons per unit volume.

Valuable information about ρ_{eh} can be obtained indirectly from CT numbers, if the data has been corrected for the variation of the mean energy of the diagnostic photon beam with depth. Furthermore, we shall assume that the computer tomograph used has been correctly calibrated to enable the conversion of CT numbers into relative electron densities.

Inhomogeneity corrections for photon beams

Three different cases have to be considered in clinical dosimetry:

Organs and tissues, including fatty tissues, the atomic composition of which is not too different from that of water and the mass density of which is near unity: between 0.92 g cm^{-3} for fat and 1.06 g cm^{-3} for muscle.

Lung which differs from soft tissues only by mass density (densities between 0.15 g cm^{-3} and 1 g cm^{-3} were measured on patients).

Bone which differs from soft tissues by mass density and by atomic composition. The mass density of cortical bone is equal to 1.85 g cm^{-3} but the average mass density of a bone as a whole varies between 1.15 and 1.65 g cm^{-3} between the various parts of the skeleton.

Sontag & Cunningham (1977) have proposed a generalised formula for tissue inhomogeneity correction based upon the Batho formulae (Batho, 1964; Young &

Gaylord, 1970), and valid for any point and any medium. They have introduced the ratio of the mean mass energy absorption coefficients between the medium r where the point lies and water to get an expression of the absorbed dose in the medium of interest. The generalised Batho formula is to be recommended for Cobalt-60 beams: it agrees within a few per cent with experimental data for any point and any biological material

$$CF = \frac{[TAR \ (d_r, A) \ ]^{(\rho_{er} - \rho_{eh})} (\bar{\mu}_{en}/\rho)_r}{[TAR \ (d_h + d_r, A)]^{(1 - \rho_{eh})} (\bar{\mu}_{en}/\rho)_w} \qquad \text{where A refers to beam size}$$

These formulae, unfortunately cannot be applied directly to very high energy photon beams (higher than a few MV) where Tissue Air Ratios (TAR) cannot be measured since they imply the measurement of a tissue absorbed dose in free air, which is the absorbed dose in an elementary mass of matter in air, the elementary mass of matter being large enough to ensure electronic equilibrium in the cavity and small enough for scattering and attenuation of photons to be negligible. For 20 MV X-rays, for instance, the minimum dimensions of this elementary mass of matter should be 4 cm of water in diameter and 5 cm in longitudinal direction (Dutreix et al, 1965). The attenuation of the photon beam can be estimated to be 15 per cent and the scattering should contribute to the dose by a few per cent in such an elementary mass.

TAR is usually replaced in clinical dosimetry by Tissue Maximum Ratio (TMR). TMR is by definition equal to 1 at the depth d_m of the maximum build-up; d_m is at most, for large distances and small field sizes equal to the maximum effective range R_e of the secondary electrons for the photon beam under consideration (Marinello & Dutreix, 1973). For small depths $(d < d_m)$ where electronic equilibrium conditions are not fulfilled, TMR is smaller than one. Then if the generalised Batho formula is used by replacing TAR by TMR it will lead to rather large errors every time the distance d_r between point Q and the interface between the two media is smaller than d_m including the case where point Q lies within the inhomogeneity $(d_r = o)$. Furthermore it is obvious that in clinical practice, on many occasions either the longitudinal or the lateral electronic equilibrium are not achieved and TMR data should only be used with caution.

Soft tissues. Let us assume that the correction factor CF is calculated in points where the electronic equilibrium is achieved, that is to say at depths greater than d_m, the depth of the maximum build-up, and for field sizes larger than $2 R_1$, where R_1 is the minimum radius ensuring lateral electronic equilibrium. It is then possible to use the Batho method when replacing TAR by TMR and adding d_m to the thicknesses in order to calculate TMR for depths larger than d_m

$$CF = \frac{[TMR \ (d_r + d_m, A) \ ]^{(\rho_{er} - \rho_{eh})}}{[TMR \ (d_h + d_r + d_m, A)]^{(1 - \rho_{eh})}}$$

Lung. As the electron density of lung is usually lower than the electron density of water, the effective range of electrons in lung expressed in centimeters is much larger than it is in water. As a first approximation the range of electrons R_h in a medium h is inversely proportional to the relative electron density ρ_{eh} of h, and proportional to the effective range in water R_w: $R_h = R_w /\rho_{eh}$. For instance, in a 25 MV X-ray beam (R_w = 5 cm), when the lung electron density is equal to 0.4, the effective range of electrons in lung is R_h = 12.5 cm and laterally R_1 = 2 cm/0.4 = 5 cm. Electron equilibrium in lung is then achieved only for a beam size larger than 2 R_1 = 10 cm and at a depth greater than 12.5 cm. It is then necessary to consider whether longitudinal and lateral electron equilibrium are achieved before choosing the best method of arriving at a correction factor.

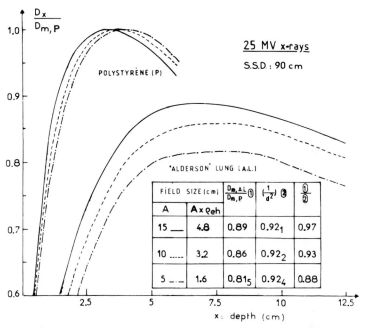

FIELD SIZE (cm)		$\frac{D_{m,AL}}{D_{m,P}}$ (1)	$(\frac{1}{d^2})$ (2)	$\frac{(1)}{(2)}$
A	A x ρ_{eh}			
15 ___	4.8	0.89	0.92₁	0.97
10	3.2	0.86	0.92₂	0.93
5 _.._	1.6	0.81₅	0.92₄	0.88

Fig. 16.1 Comparison of build-up curves measured in polystyrene and in lung equivalent material for three different field sizes 5 cm x 5 cm, 10 cm x 10 cm and 15 cm x 15 cm in a 25 MV X-ray beam.

Figure 16.1 shows build-up curves measured in a lung equivalent material (ρ_{eh} = 0.32) as compared to similar curves in polystyrene for three different field sizes (Hanna, 1979). The last column in the inserted table shows that the maximum dose (after inverse law correction) is smaller than the maximum absorbed dose in polystyrene by 3 to 12 per cent depending upon the field size because of the lack of lateral electron equilibrium.

Figure 16.2 shows the variation of the measured correction factor with depth, when a 15 cm thickness of lung equivalent material is irradiated in a 10 x 10 cm beam, behind a thickness of soft tissue d_a varying from 1 to 4 cm. The correction factor is equal to or larger than 1 at depths d_h in lung large enough for the longitudinal electronic equilibrium to be achieved. $d_h \geqslant (d_m - d_a) \cdot \rho_{ea}/\rho_{eh}$. At smaller depths, the correction factor CF is smaller than 1, that is to say that the absorbed dose in lung is lower than it would be in water.

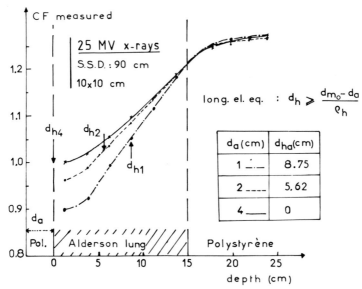

Fig. 16.2 Variation of the correction factor (CF) for 15 cm of lung equivalent material placed at a depth d_a in polystyrene of 1, 2 or 4 cm. The longitudinal electron equilibrium (CF = 1) is restored at depths d_h in lung.

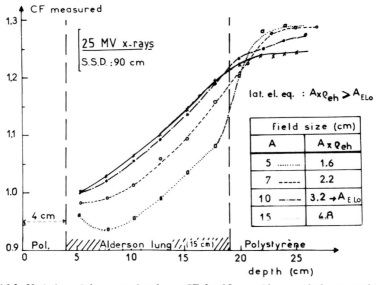

Fig. 16.3 Variation of the correction factor CF for 15 cm of lung equivalent material placed at a depth equal to 4 cm of polystyrene for four different field sizes 5 cm x 5 cm, 7 cm x 7 cm, 10 cm x 10 cm and 15 cm x 15 cm. For small field sizes, CF is lower than 1 in the first centimeters of lung due to the lack of lateral electronic equilibrium.

Figure 16.3 shows the variation of CF for various field sizes, when electronic equilibrium is achieved in soft tissue in front of the lung. For small field sizes, as the lateral electronic equilibrium is not achieved in lung, the correction factor decreases in the first few centimeters of lung and is larger than one at depths in lung greater than 9 cm and 14 cm for field sizes of 7 cm x 7 cm and 5 cm x 5 cm respectively. Empirical methods for arriving at CF in good agreement with measured values have been proposed by considering whether both the longitudinal and the lateral electron equilibrium are achieved or not at the level of the point Q under consideration. In clinical practice we shall assume that field sizes are always large enough to ensure electronic equilibrium in soft tissues. The methods are as follows:

When longitudinal electronic equilibrium is achieved ($d_x = \Sigma \rho_{ei} \cdot d_i \geqslant d_m$) and lateral electronic equilibrium is achieved ($A.\rho_{eh} \geqslant 2\ R_1$): use the corrected Batho method

$$CF = \frac{[TMR\ (d_r + d_m, A)\quad]^{(\rho_{er}\ \rho_{eh})}}{[TMR\ (d_h + d_r + d_m, A)]^{(1 - \rho_{eh})}}$$

assuming the ratio of the mean mass energy absorption coefficients is equal to 1 between lung and soft tissues.

When longitudinal electron equilibrium is achieved ($d_x = \Sigma \rho_{ei} \cdot d_i \geqslant d_m$) and lateral electron equilibrium is not achieved in lung ($A.\rho_{eh} < 2\ R_1$ and point Q lies in lung $d_r = o$), as $TMR\ (d_r + d_m) = 1$, $CF = [TMR(d_m + d_h, A) \cdot K_e]^{(\rho_{eh}-1)}$ where K_e is a coefficient taking account of the lack of lateral electronic equilibrium and calculated from build-up measurements in narrow beams in water equivalent material (Fig. 16.4) (Dutreix et al, 1965).

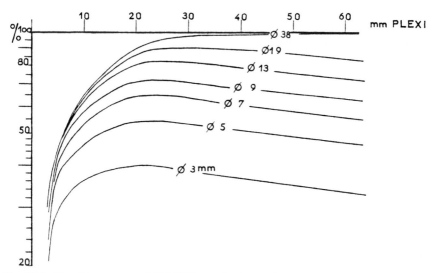

Fig. 16.4   Transition curves of 20 MV X-rays for beam diameters ranging from 3 to 38 mm. Depth dose curves are measured by film dosimetry in lucite and corrected for inverse square law and for the exponential attentuation of the photon beam.

When longitudinal electronic equilibrium is not achieved ($d_x = \Sigma \rho_{ei} \cdot d_i < d_m$), point Q lies in lung and lateral electronic equilibrium is achieved ($A.\rho_{eh} \geqslant 2\ R_1$) (we shall assume that longitudinal equilibrium is always achieved for points lying in soft tissues behind lung), in our experience the Batho method cannot be used but the simple TMR method leads to results in good agreement with measurements.

$$CF = \frac{TMR\,(d_a + \rho_{eh} \cdot d_h, A)}{TMR(d_a + d_h, A)}$$

We should note that $TMR(d_a + \rho_{eh} \cdot d_h, A)$ is much lower than 1, since $d_a + \rho_{eh} \cdot d_h < d_m$ then $CF < 1$.

When neither longitudinal nor lateral electronic equilibrium are achieved, special measurements are necessary in the irradiation conditions in order to take account of the contamination by external electrons and no formula is proposed.

Bone. The absorbed dose in soft tissues near a bone interface is increased by the increased fluence of the secondary electrons set in motion in bone. The magnitude of this dose increase cannot be easily predicted and accurate measurements or Monte-Carlo calculations would be necessary to determine the value of CF for points lying at distance d_h from a bone interface smaller than d_m/ρ_{eh}. For points at larger distances the corrected Batho method may be used.

$$CF = \frac{[TMR(d_r + d_m, A)]^{(\rho_{er} - \rho_{eh})}}{[TMR(d_h + d_r + d_m, A)]^{(1 - \rho_{eh})}} \cdot \frac{(\bar{\mu}_{en}/\rho)_r}{(\bar{\mu}_{en}/\rho)_w}$$

Inhomogeneity corrections in photon beams

In electron beams, the dose variation with depth is not exponential and there is no simple method to determine a correction factor to be applied to in-water dose distribution to take into account inhomogeneities. When a tumour is treated with an electron beam, the electron energy is usually adjusted to the maximum depth of the tumour. This electron energy is in general chosen so that the dose at the deepest limit of the target volume be equal to 80 or 85 per cent of the maximum dose in order to reduce the dose inhomogeneity throughout the target volume. The dose delivered to the healthy tissues deeper than the tumour is much lower than the tumour dose because of the high dose gradient in the last part of electron depth dose curves. When irradiated tissues are not strictly water equivalent two types of correction have to be performed. First, and by far the most important one is that the electron energy has to be modified in order to ensure a high enough dose to the deepest part of the tumour and low enough to the healthy structures deeper than the tumour; and second, the dose distribution to the deep healthy structures has to be corrected to take into account tissue inhomogeneities.

Table 16.1 Relative dose in electron beams at the deepest part of a tumour as compared with the minimum dose assumed (80 per cent). The total water-equivalent depth is underestimated by Δx

E_e (MeV)	$\Delta x = -0.5$ cm (%)	$\Delta x = -1$ cm (%)
8	50	20
10	55	35
19	66	58
25	74.5	67.5
32	76.5	72

Table 16.1 shows the relative dose at the deepest part of a tumour when the total water-equivalent thickness is underestimated by 0.5 or 1 cm. This underestimation

Δx is equal to the difference between the thicknesses x_i of tissues in centimeters corrected for the relative electron densities ρ_{ei} of the various tissues and the total thickness x in centimeters $\Delta x = \Sigma \rho_{ei} x_i - x$. To correct the treatment plan, the radiotherapist has to increase the electron energy which was planned from the in-water dose distribution. The required increase in energy ΔE is at a first approximation equal to ΔE (MeV) $= 3\Delta x$(cm). When the energy is conveniently adjusted it is necessary to correct the whole dose distribution if an accurate dose determination to healthy structures is needed.

Conclusion

CT offers a great potential for improving radiation therapy through accurate localisation of tumour and critical normal structures. However the improvement brought by more accurate inhomogeneity corrections is more controversial. Clinical experience throughout the world has been gained with in-water dose distributions. Tumour doses stated in the literature are tumour doses in error by a few per cent because of the non water-equivalence of tissues. Performing inhomogeneity corrections without clear warning for the radiotherapist in charge of the patients could lead to failure to control the patient's disease because of systematic overdosage or underdosage depending on the tissue densities in the region of interest. In the publication of doses and cure rates in clinical journals, clear statements are essential on the inhomogeneity corrections performed. Comparisons with in-water doses should be recommended during a transitional period. However refusing to perform corrections when the necessary data and methods are available would be against progress. Such corrections vary evidently for the same type of tumour from one patient to the next depending upon the depth of the tumour and the amount of fat tissues. The analysis of clinical results as a function of uncorrected doses may be erroneous because of the blurring of any small variation in local tumour control or normal tissue damage with dose. By improving dose calculations, then, one can expect to learn more accurately the dose-response and dose time-volume relationships.

References

Batho H F 1964 Lung corrections in cobalt 60 beam therapy. Journal of the Canadian Association of Radiology 15: 79-83

Dutreix J, Dutreix A, Tubiana M 1965 Electronic equilibrium and transition stages. Physics in Medicine and Biology 10: 177-190

Hanna T 1979 Performances d'un tomodensitometre. Application a son utilisation pour la correction de dose en presence d'heterogeneites dans un faisceau de photons de haute energie. Theses Universite Paul Sabatier Toulouse

Marinello G, Dutreix A 1973 Etude dosimetrique d'un faisceau de rayons X de 25 MV. Journal de Radiologie et d'Electrologie 54: 951-958

Sontag M R, Cunningham J R Corrections to absorbed dose calculations for tissue inhomogeneities. Medical Physics 4: 431-436

Young M E J, Gaylord J D 1970 Experimental tests of correction for tissue inhomogeneities in radiotherapy. British Journal of Radiology 43: 349-355

17. Alternative tomographic systems for radiotherapy planning

S. WEBB and M. O. LEACH

In recent times much importance is being ascribed to the use of cross sectional images, reconstructed from transmission X-ray projections, in the correction of radiotherapy treatment plans to take account of the presence of tissue inhomogeneities. Until such sectional information became available, simple inhomogeneity corrections were employed based on equivalent radiological path length deduced either from conventional tomograms or from AP and lateral X-ray pictures. With the advent of CT scanners the input data for more sophisticated algorithms has become available and justifies the implementation of these algorithms in treatment planning computer software. In particular Webb & Fox (1980) have shown that tissue inhomogeneity corrections with an accuracy of better than 3 per cent are obtained using a power law tissue-air ratio formula with a two dimensional map of linear attenuation coefficient as input data. The principal conclusion of their work is that this algorithm is applicable even when the lateral extent of inhomogeneities becomes smaller than the beam area; the algorithm is currently being implemented in the treatment planning programs associated with the EMI CT5005 scanner at the Royal Marsden Hospital, Sutton.

There is however evidence to suggest that the spatial resolution and resolution in linear attenuation coefficient of most commercial CT scanners is greater than is required to correct for the presence of tissue inhomogeneities (Webb et al, 1979). In certain circumstances, e.g. the localisation of lung contours, simpler CT scans would prove adequate. Additionally, it is often necessary to scan a patient in a position requiring a larger field of view than some current CT scanners provide. Thirdly, pressure on a busy department may mean a patient who would benefit from CT planned therapy may not be accommodated. There is then a case for the development of an alternative simpler CT scanner to be used in parallel with a commercial scanner within a department. Two simple scanners have been built at the Royal Marsden Hospital, Sutton, and are described in this chapter. They are both modifications of conventional equipment which possess two arms capable of rotating about a fixed axis. A Phillips simulator and a J & P Engineering double headed isotope scanner have been utilised. A simulator similar to that used will be found in most departments of radiotherapy and the modifications described enable patient cross sectional data and conventional treatment parameters such as outline to be obtained on the same machine. The patient can lie in the treatment position and without bolus. For the hospital with no commercial CT scanner a system such as this, which is capable of generating gross internal anatomical data at relatively low cost, has obvious advantages.

Computed tomography using a modified radiotherapy simulator

A radiotherapy simulator was modified to record X-ray transmission projections on film. A 100 kVp X-ray beam was collimated to a narrow fan spanning the object and defining the section to be reconstructed. The transmitted X-ray fan impinged on an X-ray film so that narrow strip shadowgraphs were recorded. In order to record a series of linear shadowgraphs on one film, the film cassette (with intensifying screens) was contained within a lead shielded guideframe with a slit aperture which corresponded with the collimated exit beam. The cassette was moved laterally within the guideframe so that sequential adjacent strips of film were exposed at each angular orientation (Fig. 17.1).

After being developed the linear shadowgraphs were processed to yield digital transmission projection data. Two data processing techniques have been employed. Early in the development of the processing facilities, films were densitised using a Joyce Loebl scanning microdensitometer connected to a graph plotter. The graphs obtained were subsequently converted to numerical data output on punched paper tape using a digitiser connected to a PDP8I computer. A more rapid technique utilised a Weston densitometer. This was automated by supplying a motor driven tray to support the film. The position of the tray was monitored via a rotational potentiometer connected by a belt to the driving motor. In this way, via an analogue to digital converter, digital film density was output to a paper tape at known linear sampling intervals. A density resolution of 0.02 was obtained and a sampling interval of 2 mm was chosen.

The difference between the film density at any particular location in a projection and the density corresponding to rays which have not passed through the body is directly proportional to the line integral of X-ray absorption along a path from the source to that location, provided both densities lie on the linear part of the film's characteristic curves. In general, measured densities fall on both knees of the curve as well as on the linear portion and the characteristic curve provides a calibrated correction rendering the density difference data truly proportional to absorption line integral. If this correction is not made a non linear reconstruction is obtained, which itself could be regarded as a processed image of the true linear reconstruction in which certain (e.g. muscle to bone) attenuation differences are suppressed whilst other (e.g. muscle to lung) attenuation differences are enhanced. Provided numerical attenuation data were not required, this contrast adjustment might even be thought desirable, particularly if lung visualisation was of special importance.

The digital projection data were submitted to an off line batch processing computer via punched cards. The data were then converted to line integral form and the two dimensional cross section was reconstructed by the convolution and back projection algorithm for divergent geometry (Lakshminarayanan, 1975) on a CDC 6600 computer at the University of London Computer Centre. The reconstructions were displayed both as lineprinter overprinted images and also as microfilm pictures with 10 levels of grey using a 64 x 64 pixel grid with a pixel size of $(5 \times 5)mm^2$. Figure 17.2 shows a reconstruction from 36 projections of a phantom prepared from muscle, lung, bone and fat substitute materials representing a 4.5 cm thick section through the 5th lumbar disk. The lung outline is apparent and an additional advantage is the simultaneous generation of the body contour.

156

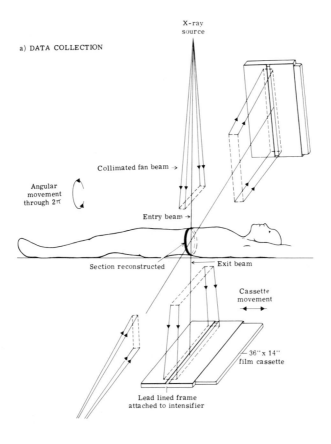

a) DATA COLLECTION

X-ray source

Collimated fan beam →

Angular movement through 2π

Entry beam →

Section reconstructed

Exit beam

Cassette movement

36" x 14" film cassette

Lead lined frame attached to intensifier

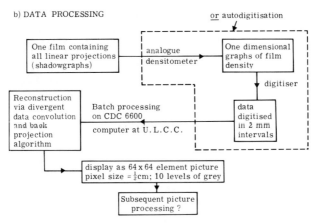

b) DATA PROCESSING

or autodigitisation

One film containing all linear projections (shadowgraphs)

analogue densitometer

One dimensional graphs of film density

digitiser

Reconstruction via divergent data convolution and back projection algorithm

Batch processing on CDC 6600 computer at U.L.C.C.

data digitised in 2 mm intervals

display as 64 x 64 element picture pixel size = ½cm; 10 levels of grey

Subsequent picture processing ?

Fig. 17.1 Geometry for computed tomography using a radiotherapy simulator and block diagram of data processing facility.

The circular boundary indicates the field of view. The reconstruction is illustrated with no modification. A smoother image was subsequently created by truncating the high frequency terms in the Fourier image and retransforming to real space.

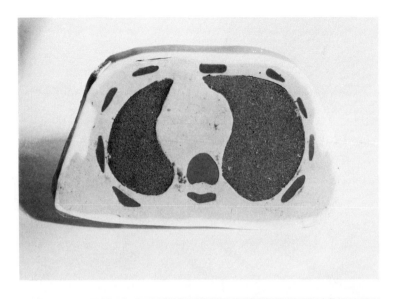

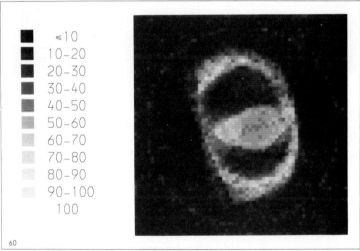

Fig. 17.2 Reconstruction of chest phantom alongside optical image of phantom (simulator scanner).

Computed tomography using a modified double headed scanner

More recently a double headed isotope scanner has been substantially modified to record transmission gamma ray projections via a completely automatic translate-rotate mode of CT data collection. This instrument enables reconstruction parameters to be quantitatively evaluated and provides a test bed convenient for developing a simple scanner for clinical use (Fig. 17.3).

158

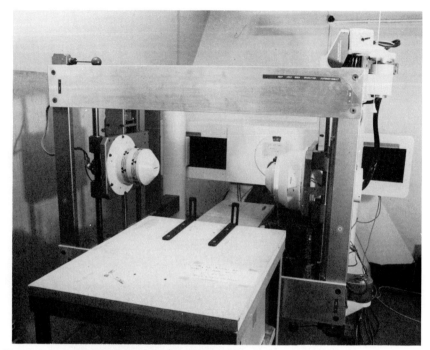

Fig. 17.3 General view of double headed scanner.

Scanner modifications

One detector head of a J & P Engineering Multipoise scanner has been completely removed and replaced by a collimated source contained in a cylindrical lead holder defining a beam of radiation of dimensions 4 cm x 2 mm and shielding the source when not in use. The source itself is ^{137}Cs pellet of activity approximately 150 mCi which is positioned parallel to the collimating slit and at 7 cm from the face of the collimator when in the 'on' position. The source can be driven from a safe position to this on position via a remote controlled servomotor (Fig. 17.4). The status of the source is indicated to the operator by a traffic light arrangement of three bulbs indicating 'safe', 'in transit' and 'on' locations. The power for the source motor is supplied independently of the main scanner.

On the other arm of the scanner the conventional focussing collimator has been replaced by a twin of the source collimator, positioned in front of the crystal/photomultiplier assembly. The two slits were optically aligned using a laser beam, with the alignment finely tuned by maximising the observed countrate. The HWHM of the radiation beam transmitted through the detector collimator was 6 mm and the detector was aligned so as to span the central 2 mm of the spread function. By disconnecting the horizontal scan drives, the two heads are permitted to scan transversely only within the plane of the section to be reconstructed.

The detector head carries a plate whose purpose is to intersect two light-beam

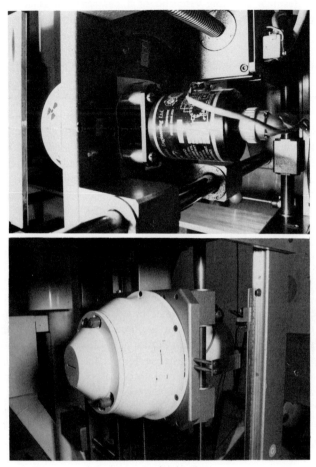

Fig. 17.4 Close up of source and detector scanning heads.

switches positioned at each end of the translational scan. These switches define the length of the transverse travel and hence the field of view. When a light beam is cut, a pulse is derived from that optical switch. The pulse provides a logic instruction to rotate the arms of the scanner to the next angular orientation and to reverse the translational motor drive for the next transverse pass in the opposite direction to that previous. The optical switches slide on a guide bar and can be repositioned before scanning to define fields of view of different area. They are however always located so that when the scanning heads are exactly midway between them, the radiation beam intersects the axis of rotation. This simplifies the organisation of the projection data prior to reconstruction.

It was observed that with no object within the field of view (i.e. an air scan) the countrate was dependent both on angular orientation and translation position. Following detailed studies, this was shown to be due to insufficient mechanical rigidity, the cone of acceptance at the detector moving with respect to the radiation cone. This variation was substantially reduced by joining the source and detector arms with two large aluminium bars and ensuring that the source is a snug fit in its holder. A residual counting variation of 8 per cent can be accommodated by correcting the projection data prior to reconstruction using a calibration derived from the air scan (see later section). The average countrate is approximately 16 k c.p.s.

A method of dynamic braking is applied to the motor controlling the angular rotation. The power is activated for a fixed time defining a fixed angular increment $S\Theta$. The fixed time may be preselected by varying a resistance in an RC timing circuit. In this way the number of parallel projections in an angular range of $O\text{-}\pi$ may be predetermined. The detector and source arms are not of equal mass and, if positioned equidistant from the axis of rotation, $S\Theta$ varies with Θ. In order to overcome this effect the two arms have been positioned so that their moments about the axis of rotation are the same, thus permitting $S\Theta$ to remain constant with respect to angle Θ. After equalisation of moments, $S\Theta$ was constant to better than 2 per cent for $O \leqslant \Theta \leqslant \pi$. As the detector arm is closer to the axis of rotation than the source arm, the field of view is presently limited to a diameter of twice the distance of the detector collimator face from the axis, rather than being limited by the distance between the optical switches.

Data collection

The output from the sodium iodide detector is passed to a single channel analyser (SCA) set to discriminate in favour of unattenuated primary photons. The SCA output pulses are input to a 24 bit counter. The counter is enabled whenever a transverse pass is in progress. A logic pulse derived from a preselected submultiple of the pulses which drive the linear scanning motors is used to gate the counter ensuring that the period between pulses corresponds to a constant distance scanned irrespective of speed. When such a logic pulse arrives, the number of counts received in the period since the arrival of the previous logic pulse is stored in the memory of an on line PDP8E computer. The counter is then zeroed and the cycle restarts. In this way, during one transverse pass of the heads, a projection is stored as a series of counts in discrete cells each corresponding to a known and fixed sampling interval. At the conclusion of each transverse scan, the projection data are output from the memory of the PDP8E to a magnetic tape cartridge via a Perex 6041 Mk III four track recorder operating in serial mode at 2400 baud. The instruction to begin data readout is the logic pulse derived from the optical switches, readout beginning after scanner rotation. When the data output is complete, acquisition of the next projection begins. The operations of translational scanning, rotation and data recording continue in this cyclic manner, without operator intervention, until a set of parallel projections in an angular range $O\text{-}\pi$ have been recorded. A range of translational speeds from 0.3 cm sec^{-1} to 1.5 cm sec^{-1} is available whilst the projection cell size can take discrete values in the range 1.3 mm to 10.4 mm. The data collection system described has recently replaced an earlier system based on the use of a multichannel analyser operating in multi-scaling mode with paper tape as the data recording medium (Webb et al, 1979).

A large computer with batch processing facilities is used for image recon-struction, display and postprocessing. The projection data is copied from the Perex cartridge tape on to 7" diameter, 9 track magnetic tape for transfer to the University of London CDC6600 computer. The data transfer from cartridge to spool tape is performed using an in house PDP11/70 computer. The magnetic tape is transferred by post to the University Computer Centre for data processing (Fig. 17.5).

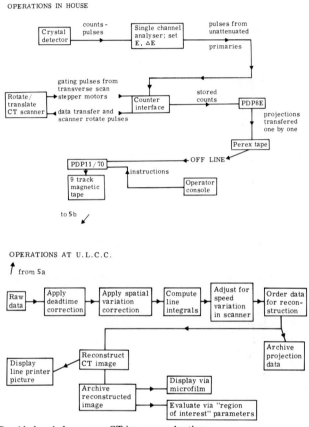

Fig. 17.5 Double headed scanner: CT image production.

Data prefiltering and CT image reconstruction, display and evaluation

Projection data prefiltering. A series of corrections to the measured projection data are necessary prior to reconstructing the cross sectional image. The corrections arise because of the inherent characteristics of the modified scanner.

Firstly the data are filtered cell by cell to correct for the counting deadtime. The deadtime for the entire system of detector, photomultiplier and counting electronics was carefully measured by counting two isotope sources first separately and then simultaneously. Solution of the quadratic equation which arises when account is taken of the background countrate yielded a value of 8 μsec for the counting deadtime.

Secondly, the data are normalised to compensate for a small difference in the speeds of translational scanning in opposite directions. Thirdly, a multiplicative correction factor is applied to each projection data point to compensate for the variation in the number of photons detected with angular orientation and translation position when no object is in the field of view. This corrects for the apparent variation in the number of photons input to each projection ray when scanning an object. The multiplicative factor was derived from calibration projection data obtained with no object in the field of view.

To derive a set of projection line integrals of X-ray linear attenuation coefficient the logarithm of the countrate in each projection cell is subtracted from the logarithm of the input countrate. Since the latter is not directly measured, the approximation is made that the observed countrate of unattenuated photons in the projection sites not corresponding to paths through the object is a measure of the input countrate at all locations. To improve statistical accuracy an average over 4N such projection sites is taken where N is the number of projections recorded. The first two and last two projection elements contribute to this average.

Finally, every alternate projection is reversed. This organises the projection data such that to the reconstruction algorithm the direction of translational scanning is always in the direction of increasing angle, Θ.

CT image reconstruction, display and evaluation. Cross sectional images have been reconstructed from the projection data using each of the better known reconstruction techniques. These are ART (Herman et al, 1973), SIRT (Gilbert, 1972), filtered back projection (Ramachandran & Lakshminarayan, 1971) and filtered back projection with variable filter cutoff (Bracewell & Riddle, 1967). The results are presented in the next section for a test object and indicate a clear preference for the latter method as the most favourable to use with this scanner. Hence, after this initial exploration, all further CT images were reconstructed by unconstrained filtered back projection with a filter whose cutoff frequency is $\frac{1}{2C} = \frac{N}{\pi D}$ where N is the number of projections, D is the diameter of the reconstruction circle and C is the reconstructed pixel size.

The CT images were displayed as lineprinter overprinted pictures and also as computer generated microfilm pictures with 10 levels of grey using a 64 x 64 grid of picture elements. Additionally via a postprocessing computer program regions of interest were selected within the image and the mean and standard deviation of the reconstructed linear attenuation coefficients was calculated. This provided parameters useful in evaluating the scanner performance. Selected line profiles may also be viewed.

A standard practice has been adopted of archiving on magnetic tape all projection data and reconstructed images, thus enabling the possibility of subsequent reviewing and image enhancement if desired. It is largely the display, image evaluation, image processing and archiving requirements which necessitate the use of a large computer at this stage. Although we are currently utilising the SNARK 75 image reconstruction package (Herman et al, 1975), the relevant subset of instructions could be implemented in house.

Reconstruction results using test phantoms

A series of CT scans has been made of the test phantom shown in Figure 17.6. The phantom is a cylindrical section of muscle equivalent material (MS11) (White et al,

1977) of diameter 24 cm containing six holes of diameters 9.1, 6.1, 3.6, 3.6, 2.3 and 0.75 cm. For some CT scans four of the holes were plugged with either lung (LN10), bone (SB5) or fat (AP3) equivalent materials. From the resulting reconstructions the means and standard deviations of the linear attenuation coefficients pertaining to the various materials in the field of view were calculated for several regions of interest. Linear attenuation coefficient is expressed in cm^{-1} with air as zero. It is however the ratio of linear attenuation coefficient for a material to that of water which is most useful (see below). The results for those regions of interest within the *same* material were then combined according to the principle of least error to yield a weighted mean together with its standard error (Barford, 1967). The weighted results are presented in Table 17.1 and in this form permit several important conclusions to be drawn. It is however important to stress that such condensed parameters for image evaluation, whilst clearly illustrating certain key dependences, can be no substitute for visually inspecting the entire reconstruction. Space limitations enable only one such reconstruction to be illustrated here (Fig. 17.6), namely that from experiment 14.

Reconstruction algorithm. Columns 1 to 4 of Table 17.1 present results for the reconstruction of the test phantom with all holes unplugged. The algorithm SIRT generates an image which although very smooth (small standard errors) gives erroneous linear attenuation coefficients. ART not only gives erroneous coefficients but is additionally very grainy (high standard errors). A better picture is obtained from the convolution and back projection algorithm with fixed cutoff $\frac{1}{2a}$ for the convolving function, where a is the projection sampling interval. Because of the mismatch of reconstruction and projection pixel sizes, however, the coefficients are not quite correct and the image is still somewhat grainy. The best image is reconstructed via the convolution and back projection algorithm with frequency cutoff $\frac{1}{2C}$. The standard errors are small and the linear attenuation coefficients are correct. Consequently this reconstruction technique was adopted for subsequent CT scans.

Dependence on counting statistics (scan time). Columns 5 and 6 of Table 17.1 illustrate results for the fastest and slowest scan modes available with the test phantom having none of its holes plugged. Similarly columns 7 and 8 correspond with the same two modes with the test phantom containing lung substitute plugs, and columns 9 and 11 are for the same two modes with the holes plugged with bone substitute material. Inspection of the standard errors illustrates clearly the expected conclusion that, with a longer scan time, the standard errors are reduced. Experiments at intermediate speeds confirm the trend. It is perhaps somewhat surprising, however, that as the scan time decreases from 145 mins to 36 mins the standard errors do not *seriously* degenerate. Inspection of the complete reconstructed images testifies to the acceptability of the 36 mins scans wherein the smallest hole of diameter 7.5 mm is still visible. Gore & Tofts (1979) have shown that the error in linear attenuation coefficient depends on the inverse square root of the total number of photons passing through the object. Their result is derived however under several limiting assumptions, namely for a uniform circular object with projections obtained using perfectly parallel geometry and perfect collimation. Predictions based upon it would not be expected to apply for a scan of a nonuniform object.

Table 17.1 Reconstructed linear attenuation coefficients illustrating key dependences

Scan number	4	4	4	4	3	14	9	15	11	11¹	13	17
Reconstruction technique	SIRT (2 iterations)	ART (4 iterations)	Ram & Lak	Bracewell	Bracewell	Bracewell	Bracewell	Bracewell	Bracewell	Bracewell	Bracewell	Bracewell
Time per CT scan (mins)	77	77	77	77	36	145	36	145	36	36	145	145
Number of projections in 0–2π	65	65	65	65	65	65	65	65	65	33	65	65
Number of recorded photons	40.3×10^6	40.3×10^6	40.3×10^6	40.3×10^6	13.2×10^6	85.8×10^6	13.8×10^6	78.1×10^6	12.9×10^6	6.4×10^6	72.7×10^6	70.6×10^6
Material												
Air	0.0273 ±0.0008	0.0209 ±0.00334	0.0000 ±0.00105	0.0004 ±0.00017	0.0026 ±0.00021	0.00026 ±0.00014	0.00026 ±0.00030	0.00013 ±0.00016	0.00039 ±0.00027	-0.00052 ±0.00014	0.00026 ±0.00022	0.00026 ±0.00018
Lung	–	–	–	–	–	–	0.0471 ±0.00025	0.0468 ±0.00019	–	–	–	–
Muscle	0.0376 ±0.00014	0.2404 ±0.00668	0.0813 ±0.00225	0.0793 ±0.00031	0.0777 ±0.00036	0.0805 ±0.00024	0.0806 ±0.00031	0.0807 ±0.00021	0.0818 ±0.00029	0.0813 ±0.00036	0.0818 ±0.00026	0.0810 ±0.00025
Bone	–	–	–	–	–	–	–	–	0.1390 ±0.00043	0.1392 ±0.00057	0.1382 ±0.00022	–
Fat	–	–	–	–	–	–	–	–	–	–	–	0.0737 ±0.00014

All CT scans were reconstructed from projections with 285 cells of size 1.3 mm

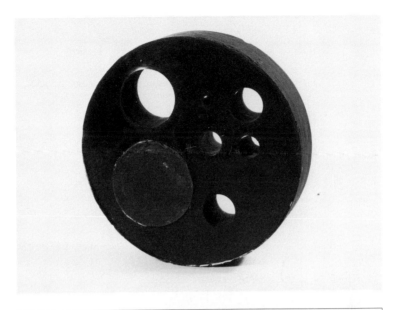

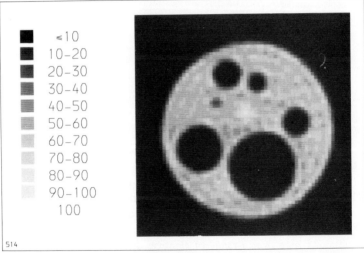

Fig. 17.6 Test phantom and reconstruction via convolution and back projection technique of Bracewell from 65 views comprising 85.8 x 10⁶ photon counts (double headed scanner).

Calibration of scanner produced linear attenuation coefficients in terms of relative electron density. The double headed CT scanner has been calibrated by scanning a phantom comprising tubes of fluids the ratio of whose electron density (electrons cm⁻³) relative to water $\left(\frac{\rho_{el}M}{\rho_{el}W}\right)$ is known. For a region of interest within each fluid the ratio $R = \left(\frac{\mu_M - \mu_A}{\mu_W - \mu_A}\right)$ was determined where μ_M is the mean linear attenuation coefficient of the fluid and μ_A and μ_W, that for air and water respectively. Additionally a CT number $H = 500 \, (R - 1)$ was determined for each calibration fluid. From Figure 17.7 it can be seen that there is a linear relationship between R (and H) and $\left(\frac{\rho_{el}M}{\rho_{el}W}\right)$ over the wide range $0 \lesssim \left(\frac{\rho_{el}M}{\rho_{el}W}\right) \lesssim 1.7$ corresponding with -500 $\leqslant H \leqslant + 350$. This indicates that within this region Compton scatter is the predomin-

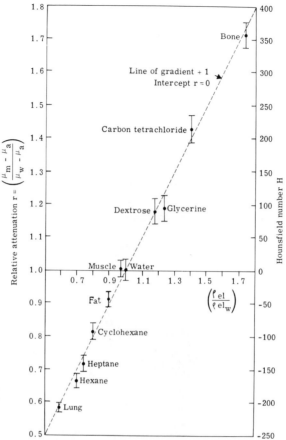

Fig. 17.7 Scanner calibration of linear attenuation coefficient vs relative electron density.

ant interaction at ^{137}Cs energy in agreement with the deductions of Webb & Parker (1978) from Monte Carlo simulations of the photon interactions in water. The linearity contrasts however with the knee seen in the equivalent calibration for the EMI CT5005 scanner operating at 140 kVp (Parker et al, 1979). The simple linearity obtained here over a range of electron densities similar to those of body tissues using a scanner operating at 662 KeV is an advantage when interpreting CT numbers for use in radiotherapy planning. The error bars in Figure 17.7 are $\pm$ 1 standard errors in $\frac{\mu_M - \mu_A}{\mu_W - \mu_A}$. In order to generate the most accurate calibration, the slowest scan time of 145 mins was employed. Additionally, the data for muscle, bone, lung and fat substitute materials has been incorporated into Figure 17.7.

Dependence on number of views. Klug & Crowther (1972) have shown that the maximum number N of projections which needs to be recorded is about $\pi/2$ times the number of cells across the reconstruction region ($N = \frac{\pi D}{2C}$). Hence to resolve a pixel of size 5 mm within the test object of diameter 24 cm, about 75 projections are needed. Operating with 65 recorded projections, the CT scans reported are close to optimum. In order to assess the degradation introduced by sub-optimal scanning a CT scan using only 33 contributing projections was performed. The results (column 10, Table 17.1) indicate the increased standard errors within the resulting image.

The spatial resolution of the scanner was estimated by reconstructing an image of a star phantom comprising twelve 15° sectors of perspex interleaved by twelve 15° sectors of air. The slowest scan time of 145 minutes yielded an image in which, within the central circle of diameter 6 cm, the image was blurred and the sectors indistinguishable. This indicates that the high contrast spatial resolution was of the order 7 mm with this scanning speed.

Body phantom. Figure 17.8 illustrates the reconstruction of the body cross section phantom described previously. 65 projections, sampled at 1.3 mm intervals and

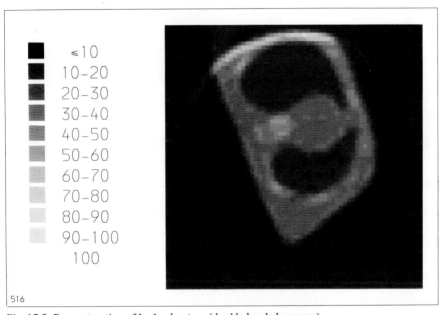

Fig. 17.8 Reconstruction of body phantom (double headed scanner).

comprising 83.5 x 10^6 photons were used. The reconstruction clearly illustrates lung contour, external outline and bones. It is an improvement over the corresponding reconstruction (Webb et al, 1979) obtained with the old data collection system and before the stabilising bars were added to the scanner.

In vivo lung imaging. A cross section, 4 cm wide, through the thorax of a rabbit has been imaged using the double headed CT scanner. The cross section was reconstructed from 65 projections samples at 1.3 mm intervals and comprising 23.4 x 10^6 photons. The complete CT scan took 36 minutes during which time the rabbit (New Zealand White, of mass 2.5 kgm was anaesthetised and exhibited shallow breathing. Figure 17.9 illustrates the 64 x 64 pixel reconstruction with a pixel size of 2.5 mm. The lungs are clearly visible. Utilising the scanner calibration in

168

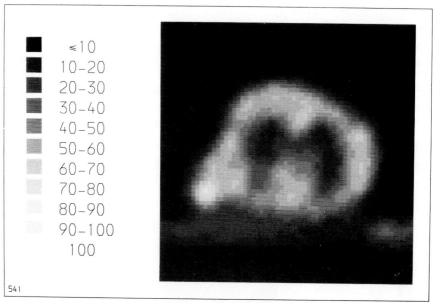

Fig. 17.9 Reconstruction of rabbit thorax.

Figure 17.7 and a region of interest situated within the lungs and comprising 72 pixels, a value for the relative attenuation of $r = \frac{\mu_{lung} - \mu_{air}}{\mu_{water} - \mu_{air}} = 0.44$ (-280 CT units) was obtained. The standard error on r was 8 CT units. The rabbit lung material in vivo appears to have a slightly, but significantly, smaller relative electron density than material LN10. However the successful delineation of the lung contour is most encouraging bearing in mind the duration of the scan, the lung movement during breathing and the width of the cross section.

Concluding remarks

It is clear that the spatial resolution and resolution of linear attenuation coefficients that can be obtained with these simplified CT devices is entirely adequate for tissue inhomogeneity correction and for the production of body contours. It is possible that devices such as those described might be suitable for construction in hospitals not possessing a diagnostic CT scanner whilst parallel development in a hospital with these facilities will free the expensive scanner for diagnostic work and complement its use for large field CT scanning. The cross sectional information obtained is suitable for interfacing with treatment planning dose calculations.

Acknowledgements

We should like to record a debt of thanks to all our colleagues in the Physics Department who have been associated with the work reported here and in particular to Drs R.E. Bentley, F. Duck, R.A. Fox, S.C. Lillicrap, J. Milan and R.D. Speller. We are also much indebted to Mr R. Kent, Mr P. Newbery,

Mr S. King, Mr H. Hodt, Mr M. Phillips and Mr P. Collins of our workshop staff for construction and helpful discussions.

References

Barford N C 1967 Experimental measurements: precision error and truth. Addison-Wesley, London, Ch 3, p 62-64

Bracewell R N, Riddle A C 1967 Inversion of fan-beam scans in radioastronomy. Astrophysical Journal 150: 427-434

Gilbert P 1972 Iterative methods for the three-dimensional reconstruction of an object from projections. Journal of Theoretical Biology 36: p 105

Gore J C, Tofts P S 1979 Statistical limitations in computed tomography. Physics in Medicine and Biology 23: 1176-1182

Herman G T, Lent A, Rowland S W 1973 ART: mathematics and applications. Journal of Theoretical Biology 42: 1-32

Herman G T, Hinds J A, Peretti R W, Rowland S W 1975 SNARK 75 - A programming system for the reconstruction of objects from shadowgraphs. State University of New York at Buffalo Department of Computer Science, Technical Report no. 96

Klug A, Crowther A 1972 Three dimensional image reconstruction from the viewpoint of information theory. Nature 238: 435-440

Lakshminarayaran A V 1975 Reconstruction from divergent ray data. State University of New York at Buffalo Department of Computer Science, Technical Report no. 92

Parker R P, Hobday P A, Cassell K J 1979 The direct use of CT numbers in radiotherapy dosage calculations for inhomogeneous media. Physics in Medicine and Biology 24 (4): 802-809

Ramachandran G N, Lakshminarayaran A V 1971 Three dimensional reconstruction from radiographs and electron micrographs – application of convolutions instead of Fourier transforms. Proceedings of the National Academy of Sciences, USA 68: 2236-2240

Webb S, Fox R A 1980 Verification by Monte Carlo methods of a power law tissue-air-ratio algorithm for inhomogeneity corrections in photon beam dose calculations. Physics in Medicine and Biology 25 (2): 225-240

Webb S, Parker R P 1978 A Monte Carlo study of the interaction of external beam X-radiation with inhomogeneous media. Physics in Medicine and Biology 23 (6): 1043-1059

Webb S, Speller R D, Leach M O 1979 The generation of CT data for radiotherapy planning using devices other than commercial scanners. Proceedings of the European Association of Radiology Workshop on Computerised Tomographic Scanners in Radiotherapy in Europe. Geneva, March 1979 British Journal of Radiology Supplement 15 (in press).

White D R, Martin R J, Darlison R 1977 Epoxy resin based tissue substitutes. British Journal of Radiology 50: 814-821

18. Quantitative tissue characterisation in CT—does it work?

R. T. RITCHINGS, B. R. PULLAN and I. ISHERWOOD

Introduction

The pictures produced by computed tomographic scanners show the spatial distribution of X-ray attenuation in a slice through the human body. While the attenuation values allow identification of the various components in the pictures, tissue type cannot always be determined, particularly in the case of disease.

Several attempts have been made to derive quantitative parameters for tissue characterisation. The approach taken is some type of analysis of the attenuation values in a small region of tissue; the size of the region usually being limited by the need to avoid artefacts. Three types of analysis have been used and these will be reviewed in this paper. These include the determination of chemical composition of tissues, the examination of the probability distribution of the attenuation values, and the statistical examination of the spatial distribution of the attenuation values.

Tissue characterisation by chemical composition

The basis of the techniques used to determine chemical composition is that in CT two processes, Compton scattering and photo-electric absorption, are responsible for the X-ray attenuation. Compton scattering is related to the density of the tissue present, while the photo-electric absorption is related to the nature of the tissue. These two processes are energy dependent; Compton scattering being predominant at the high X-ray energies, and the approach usually taken to try and separate the attenuation due to these processes involves scanning the patient at two or more X-ray energies.

Three methods have been used to take scans at different energies. The simplest one is to take separate scans at the different X-ray energies. Many studies of brain lesions were made using this technique (Rutherford et al, 1976; McDavid et al, 1977; Dubal and Wiggli, 1977; Marshall et al, 1977; Latchaw et al, 1978). The main problem is that of patient movement between the scans. While this may not be too severe for brain studies, the problems increase with physiological movements in the body. Another approach is to develop detectors which are sensitive to more than one X-ray energy (Brooks & Di Chiro, 1978; Fenster, 1978). This requires considerable modification to the X-ray scanners and few results have yet been seen. A more recent approach has involved filtering half of the X-ray beam by placing tin foil over half of the detectors (Ritchings & Pullan, 1979). Using this technique, the mean energy of the photons passing through the foil is raised by the well-known 'beam-hardening' process, while the unfiltered beam has the usual lower X-ray energy. This approach is simple to implement; the only requirements are a hardware modification to the detector collimator, and a software program to separate the 'dual energy' projection data prior to the standard picture processing.

Various computational methods have been used to derive chemical composition of tissues from dual energy scans (Rutherford et al, 1976; Latchaw et al, 1978; Brooks, 1977). Information can be presented as two pictures, one showing the effective atomic number (usually labelled Z^*) and another one showing either the effective atomic density (usually labelled n^*) or the effective electron density (usually labelled ρ_e^*).

The chemical composition of several types of brain lesion has been determined (Rutherford et al, 1976; McDavid et al, 1977; Dubal & Wiggli, 1977; Marshall et al, 1977; Latchaw et al, 1978) and preliminary results are now available on studies of trabecular bone using the filter technique (Adams et al, 1980). These methods do not appear at present, however, to have a general role in the characterisation of tissue.

Tissue characterisation using the probability distribution of attenuation values

The attenuation values represent the mean X-ray attenuation in a small volume, or voxel, of tissue. In a uniform region of tissue, the attenuation values will not be identical but symmetrically distributed about a mean value, largely due to statistical fluctuations in the attenuation process. The basis of the approach to tissue characterisation described in this section is that disease might produce a slight change in the probability distribution of the attenuation values.

The probability distribution can be described by a histogram of attenuation values. Changes in the shape of the histogram due to disease may be a shift to higher or lower attenuation values or an increase or decrease in the width of the histogram. These two effects may be quantified by calculating the mean value and standard deviation of the attenuation values respectively.

The measurements have been made for normal and atrophied brains (Pullan et al, 1978) and normal and cirrhotic livers (Ritchings et al, 1979). Neither the mean values nor the standard deviations have been found to be statistically different for the normal and diseased tissues. Higher order statistics, such as the skewness of the distribution, have also been examined but proved unsuccessful in separating tissue types. The probability distribution of attenuation values, therefore, has not so far been of value in providing unique characterisation studies.

Tissue characterisation using the spatial distribution of attenuation values

Some tissue characterisation has been obtained from statistical studies of the spatial distribution of the attenuation values (Pullan et al, 1978; Ritchings et al, 1979). Two types of analysis have been made in order to quantify spatial structure in a region of tissue. These are an autocorrelation analysis and an analysis of the magnitude and directions of the gradients.

The autocorrelation technique basically produces a measure of the tendency for attenuation values separated by a particular number of picture elements, or pixels,

172

to have similar or correlated values. The degree of correlation is usually calculated for several pixel separations and plotted in graphical form as shown in Figure 18.1 (Ritchings et al, 1979). In the case of CT scans of liver, these graphs, when

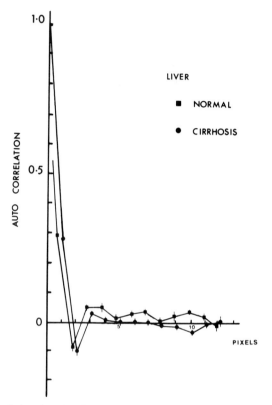

Fig. 18.1 Autocorrelation function for normal and cirrhotic liver, taken from Ritchings et al, 1979.

calculated for normal and cirrhotic patients, have been found to be significantly different for both a preliminary sample (Pullan et al, 1978) and a further definitive group of patients. The difference in the graphs is very small (Fig. 18.1) with the major separation being at about 10 pixels. The cause of the small structural difference between normal and cirrhotic liver was not established by the authors and could represent either a genuine pathological change or possibly an effect due to varying movement during the scan, a feature which itself might be associated with the disease process. This approach, nevertheless, does seem to be of value in distinguishing cirrhosis from normal liver.

The gradient's analysis determines the maximum gradient, or slope at each point in the region, and examines the probability distribution of the magnitudes of these gradients. As in the case of the probability distribution of attenuation values, no significant differences were found between normal and diseased tissue (Pullan et al, 1978).

Promising results, however, were obtained by these authors from studies of the directions of the gradients. If the sample region is uniform, the attenuation values should be random numbers with a probability distribution quantified by the mean and standard deviation of the attenuation values discussed in the previous section. In such a situation, the directions of the gradients would be equally distributed between 0 and 180 degrees. The effect of structure in the region would be to change the uniformity of the angular distribution.

A measurement of the non-uniformity of the angular distribution of the gradients can be obtained from the X^2 value which is given by

$$X^2 = \frac{[E(\Theta)\,\delta\,\Theta - O\,(\Theta)\,\delta\Theta]^2}{E(\Theta)\delta\Theta}$$

In this equation $O(\Theta)\delta\Theta$ and $E(\Theta)\delta\Theta$ are the observed and expected number of gradients in the range of angles Θ to $\Theta+\delta\Theta$ respectively, and for the expected uniform distribution of N elements $E(\Theta)\delta\Theta = N\frac{\delta\Theta}{360}$. The angular interval, $\delta\Theta$, chosen for the study was such that there were 10 intervals between 0 and 180 degrees. The gradients and their directions need not be calculated from adjacent pixels. In the preliminary study these parameters were calculated over a range of distances and the results presented as a graph showing the variation of X^2 with the distance over which the gradients were calculated. The preliminary results are shown in Figure 18.2 for patients with normal and atrophied brains, and a significant difference can be seen between the two graphs. The preliminary trial was made

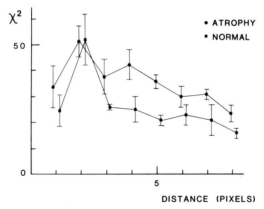

Fig. 18.2 X^2 as a function of distance for normal and atrophied brain, taken from Pullan et al, 1978.

on four normal patients and four showing atrophy, using an early water bath brain scanner (CT1000). A larger study has recently been made using the EMI CT5005 general purpose scanner in the University Department of Diagnostic Radiology. It has not been possible to repeat the initial results.

A reappraisal of the second set of data has been made and it appears that the failure to reproduce these earlier results might be a consequence of employing a general purpose scanner rather than a water bath brain scanner. The brain scanner used in the successful preliminary trial was inherently better calibrated and more

174

sensitive. It is suggested, therefore, that the higher noise levels in the general purpose scanner (a factor of 2 for a slow scan) served to obscure the small structural change in brain tissue observed earlier.

In order to justify this conclusion, the gradients' directions analysis has been performed on water scans from both the early water bath scanner and the general purpose scanner. The individual graphs of X^2 against distance for four adjacent regions are shown in Figure 18.3A for the water bath scanner, and Figure 18.3B for the general purpose scanner. The fluctuations seen in Figure 18.3B are clearly much greater than in Figure 18.3A and comparable with the separation between the results for normal and atrophied brains seen in Figure 18.2. In view of the noise

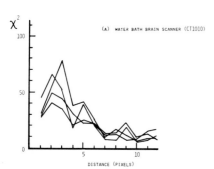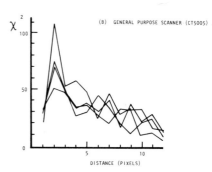

Fig. 18.3 X^2 as a function of distance for four adjacent regions of a water scans taken on (A) an early water bath brain scanner (CT1000) and (B) a general purpose scanner (CT5005).

levels in Figure 18.3B, it is not surprising that this type of separation was not observed in the recent study. The results of the preliminary trial are thus still unconfirmed, and it seems that a CT machine with lower noise than the present general purpose scanner will be required.

Conclusion

Tissue characterisation studies have been of limited value to date. Only in the case of normal and cirrhotic livers has a preliminary result been confirmed by a later study. The failure to reproduce the preliminary separation of normal and atrophied brains, emphasises the need for well calibrated scanners with low noise levels.

At present, the evidence suggests that tissue characterisation can work in some situations, but is dependent on the sensitivity of the CT scanner used.

Acknowledgements

We would like to thank Mr Ian Foy for the preparation of the illustrative material and Mrs Peggy Burt for her secretarial assistance.

References

Adams J E, Isherwood I, Ritchings R T, Pullan B R, Adams P H 1980 The estimation of bone mass in vitro using CT scanning ESCAT 2

Brooks R A 1977 A quantitative theory of the Hounsfield unit and its application to dual energy scanning. Journal of Computer Assisted Tomography 1: 487-493

Brooks R A, Di Chiro G 1978 Split-detector CAT — a preliminary report. Radiology 126: 255

Dubal L, Wiggli U 1977 Tomochemistry of the brain. Journal of Computer Assisted Tomography 1: 300-307

Fenster A 1978 Split xenon detector for tomochemistry in computed tomography. Journal of Computer Assisted Tomography 2: 243-252

Latchaw R E, Payne J T, Gold L H A 1978 Effective atomic number and electron density as measured with a computed tomography scanner: computation and correlation with brain tumor histology. Journal of Computer Assited Tomography 2: 199-208

McDavid W D, Waggener R G, Dennis M J, Sank V J, Payne W H 1977 Estimation of chemical composition and density from computed tomography carried out at a number of energies. Investigative Radiology 12: 189-194

Marshall W H Jr, Easter W, Zatz L M 1977 Analysis of the dense lesion at computed tomography with dual kVp scans. Radiology 124: 87-89

Pullan B R, Fawcitt R, Isherwood I 1978 Tissue characterisation by an analysis of the distribution of attenuation values in CT scans: a preliminary report. Journal of Computer Assisted Tomography 2: 49-54

Ritchings R T, Pullan B R 1979 A technique for simultaneous dual energy scanning. Journal of Computer Assisted Tomography 3(6): 842-846

Ritchings R T, Pullan B R, Lucas S B, Fawcitt R A, Best J J K, Isherwood I, Morris A I 1979 An analysis of the spatial distribution of attenuation values in computed tomographic scans of liver and spleen. Journal of Computer Assisted Tomography 3(1): 36-39

Rutherford R A, Pullan B R, Isherwood I 1976 Measurements of effective atomic number and electron density using an EMI scanner. Neuroradiology 11: 15-21

19. Quantitation of therapeutic response

JANET HUSBAND, PAULINE HOBDAY and K. J. CASSELL.

The ability to document tumour regression and regrowth has obvious application to patient management and important biological significance for the study of human tumour behaviour. The rapid development of imaging techniques during recent years has provided much information which has hitherto been impossible to obtain, thus permitting an opportunity to study the response of tumours to treatment. These imaging techniques fall into two major categories: those which depend on the physical characteristics of the system to demonstrate abnormalities and those which depend on physiological mechanisms so that a lesion is shown on account of its abnormal function. The first group which may be regarded as anatomical, includes conventional radiology, ultrasound and computed tomography. The second group includes thermography and isotope scanning. Using these imaging techniques information can be obtained regarding the size, composition and function of tumours and it follows that changes in one or more of these parameters may be used to assess therapeutic response. In practical terms alteration in tumour size is the most widely used, partly because it is generally accepted that tumour shrinkage indicates response to treatment and partly because change in tumour size is frequently the only parameter which is measurable.

This paper discussed the role of computed tomography as a method of monitoring therapeutic response. Using this technique, changes in tumour size can be elegantly displayed and in certain tumours, changes in composition may also be appreciated. At the Royal Marsden Hospital, approximately 1400 body CT examinations are carried out annually and of these, approximately 500 are repeat scans. This illustrates the importance of CT for monitoring therapeutic response of tumours in the chest, abdomen and pelvis. In this review the use of CT will be considered for studying growth and regression of pulmonary metastases and for deep-seated abdominal tumours according to the parameters of tumour volume and tumour composition.

Pulmonary metastases

Volume

The greatest amount of published work on the growth of human tumours has been obtained from observations on pulmonary metastases using conventional radiology (Collins et al, 1956; Breur et al, 1965). This is because the majority of pulmonary metastases can be clearly delineated on the plain chest radiograph. Pulmonary metastases are surrounded by homogeneous tissue and can grow freely in all directions. They are therefore assumed to be spherical and calculations of tumour volume can be made. From such observations, growth curves for pulmonary metastases have been produced and there is now sufficient evidence to indicate that the growth of pulmonary metastases is predominantly exponential (Steel & Lamerton, 1966).

The accuracy of measuring pulmonary metastases on the plain chest radiograph can only be examined by correlation of radiographic observations with the size of lesions removed at thoracotomy or at post mortem examinations. Few such studies have been reported but Spratt & Spratt (1964) showed good correlation between the size of pulmonary metastases measured at post mortem and the size of the metastases extrapolated from radiographic observations in 118 patients. Thus, in the majority of patients a plain chest film appears to be an accurate method of assessing tumour growth and regression. Furthermore, since the technique causes little inconvenience to the patient, it can be repeated frequently at low cost. However, there are several disadvantages of conventional chest radiography. In certain tumour types, such as carcinoma of the breast, the metastases tend to be ill-defined and are therefore unsuitable for measurement. Normal structures such as ribs, hila, heart or diaphragm, may obscure the margin of a metastasis preventing visualisation. Similarly, metastases may be hidden by an area of consolidation or fibrosis. One of the major limitations of plain chest film is the inability to define metastases less than 1 cm in diameter and thus information on growth curves of pulmonary metastases in the silent interval before metastases can be recognised is lacking.

Computed tomography demonstrates the lungs in the cross-sectional plane unobscured by the chest wall and mediastinum. Hence, lesions can be seen in those sites which are difficult or impossible to assess on the plain chest radiograph and in addition metastases as small as 2 to 3 mm in diameter can be detected at the lung periphery (Fig. 19.1). CT scanning may therefore be used for assessing response or growth of a large metastasis obscured on a plain chest film and this is particularly important if the metastasis is solitary (Fig. 19.2). CT may also be valuable for studying those metastases which are too small to be examined by conventional radiology and from such observations studies on the growth of pulmonary metastases in the 'silent interval' or 'pre-clinical phase' may be obtained.

Composition

In general, both conventional radiology and CT do not provide information regarding changes in the composition of pulmonary metastases in response to treatment. A rare example is illustrated in Figure 19.3. This patient developed pulmonary metastases from testicular teratoma and was treated with chemotherapy for six months. A follow-up chest film showed no abnormality indicating tumour regression to a size below that which could be detected by conventional techniques. However, CT examinations of the lungs carried out during this remission showed several cavities each with a well-defined thin wall (Fig. 19.3). These cavities almost certainly represented the residual metastases because the patient subsequently relapsed with multiple metastases in those sites where the cavities have been demon-

178

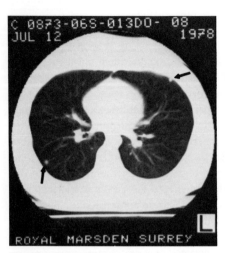 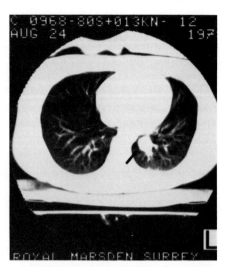

Fig. 19.1 (left) CT scan of the chest showing two pulmonary metastases, each less than 1 cm in diameter (arrowed).
Fig. 19.2 (right) CT scan of the chest showing a solitary metastasis situated behind the left heart border (arrowed). This metastasis measures 2 cm in diameter.

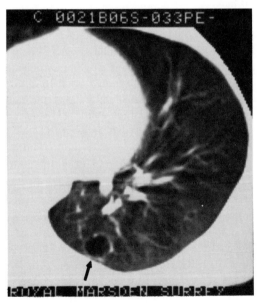

Fig. 19.3 Enlarged quadrant of a CT scan of the chest showing a cavity in the posterior aspect of the left lung (arrowed). The cavity represents a residual metastasis and has a well-defined wall.

strated. Thus, in this patient there had been a change in composition of the original pulmonary deposits rather than a significant change in tumour size.

Abdominal tumours

Volume

Conventional radiology has only a limited role in the evaluation of therapeutic response of abdominal and pelvic masses because many tumours cannot be adequately demonstrated. However, useful information has been obtained regarding regression and regrowth of tumours in such sites as the bowel (Welin et al, 1963) and lymph nodes (Macdonald et al, 1968; Haefliger et al, 1979). CT scanning has the advantage over conventional radiology that tumours can be shown without the use of contrast medium; it is therefore possible to demonstrate tumours in those sites which are inaccessible using conventional radiology and to show the full extent of masses which are only partly visualised on conventional abdominal films.

At the Royal Marsden Hospital approximately one-third of the body CT examinations are carried out to monitor therapeutic response. In the majority of these patients the assessment is subjective rather than quantitative. There are three main reasons for adopting a subjective approach. Firstly, accurate measurement of changes in tumour volume are not possible in many tumours, due to the difficulty in defining the tumour margin. Secondly, accurate tumour volume measurements is a time-consuming procedure which at the present time can only be undertaken as a research investigation. Thirdly, subjective assessment of the change in tumour size often provides adequate information for management of an individual patient (Figs. 19.4A and 4B). However, in selected patients quantitative assessment of tumour volume is feasible. Tumour volume calculations are made using one of the

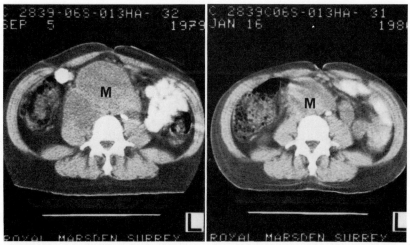

Fig. 19.4A CT scan through the fourth lumbar vertebra showing a large abdominal nodal mass (M) in a patient with a testicular teratoma. This CT examination was carried out before chemotherapy was commenced.

Fig. 19.4B CT scan through the fourth lumbar vertebra in the same patient following four courses of chemotherapy. There is obvious regression of the abdominal mass (M).

facilities available on the EMIPLAN 7000 System. CT scan data are transferred from the EMI General Purpose Scanner (CT5005) to a floppy disc and then to a cartridge disc in the EMIPLAN equipment. The CT image is displayed on the video monitor and the tumour is then outlined using a precision touch sensitive light pen (Fig. 19.5). The area within the outline is calculated by the tumour volume

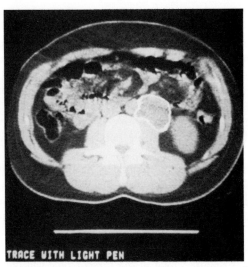

Fig. 19.5 CT scan showing a large abdominal nodal mass in a patient with a testicular teratoma. The area of the tumour has been outlined using the precision touch-sensitive light pen.

programme from the number and size of picture elements (pixels) within the outline. The procedure is repeated on adjacent slices throughout the tumour length and the final tumour volume is then calculated from the areas outlined, the slice thickness and the inter-slice intervals. The method has previously been described in more detail (Husband et al, 1980). Intrinsic errors of the method include the algorithm used, the pixel size and the observer's ability to reproduce the tumour outline. When attempting to measure human tumours further errors are incurred which relate to the difficulty of defining the precise tumour margin. Clearly, certain tumours are easier to outline than others depending on the difference in density between the tumour and the background.

The accuracy of tumour volume estimations in vivo can only be assessed by comparing the CT volume with the volume of the tumour excised at surgery or at post mortem examination. Such information is still insufficient to make conclusive statements but early work in our department has indicated good correlation. The intrinsic accuracy of the method has been tested by scanning potatoes in a water bath. These results indicate that the errors are considerably less than 10 per cent (Husband et al, 1980).

Tumour volume estimations have been performed in a group of patients with abdominal nodal metastases from testicular teratomas. This tumour type has been studied because retroperitoneal nodal masses are clearly delineated with CT and also because the volume of metastatic disease influences prognosis (Tyrrell &

Peckham, 1976). Figure 19.6 demonstrates the results of tumour volume regression in 10 patients who were treated with chemotherapy. Tumour volume has been expressed as a percentage of the initial absolute tumour volume for clear representation.

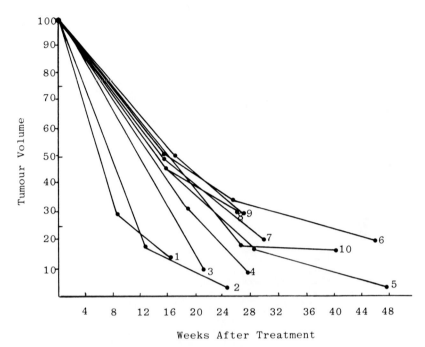

Fig. 19.6   Tumour volume regression rates in 10 patients treated with chemotherapy for abdominal nodal metastases from testicular teratoma. Tumour volume is shown on the ordinate as a percentage of the initial absolute volume (range 20-1200 cc).

In order to assess the accuracy of subjective CT reporting, CT volume calculations were compared with visual CT reporting in 22 patients. The results are shown in Table 19.1 and indicate that subjective reporting is frequently inaccurate.

Table 19.1   Correlation of visual and quantitative estimations of tumour volume

Visual		Quantitative	
CT Report		Increase	Decrease
No change	9	5	4
Regression	13	–	13
Total	22	5	17

In 9 patients quantitative estimations of tumour volume indicated significant regression or regrowth which had not been appreciated by visual reporting. (The percentage change by quantitative assessment ranged from 20 to 80 per cent of the initial absolute volume − range 20 to 150 ml).

Tumour composition

As in the lungs changes in composition of tumours in the abdomen are rarely appreciated with CT except occasionally in the brain and liver. Figures 19.7A, 7B and 7C illustrate changes in tumour composition (CT number) which occurred in a patient with liver metastases from carcinoid syndrome. Following the initial CT scan (Fig. 19.7A) therapeutic embolisation of the liver was undertaken in order

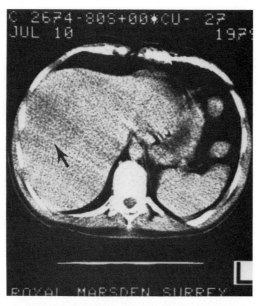

Fig. 19.7A   CT scan through the liver in a patient with carcinoid syndrome. After injection of intravenous contrast medium a low density area is visible in the right lobe of the liver (arrowed). This lesion is not well shown because the attenuation values are close to that of normal liver.

to relieve severe symptoms. Repeat CT examination after an interval of three weeks clearly demonstrated that the lesions had become cystic (Fig. 19.7B). Three months later, the patient's symptoms recurred and a CT examination carried out at this time showed that the metastases were similar in appearance to the original scan, i.e. the attenuation values had increased (Fig. 19.7C). These changes in tumour composition almost certainly represent response to treatment and subsequent tumour regrowth. However, quantitative CT number data is subject to several sources of error of which the most important are photon and scan noise. Other errors are due to variation of position, size and shape of the object and artefacts. In the measurement of human tumours streak artefacts from movement or from the structures of high density (e.g. bone) increase the errors of measurement. The magnitude of these errors is difficult to assess when attempting to quantitate CT number changes in human tumours in response to treatment and it is difficult at the present time to make conclusive statements. Further work is clearly required to establish the biological significance of any CT number changes recorded in this paper.

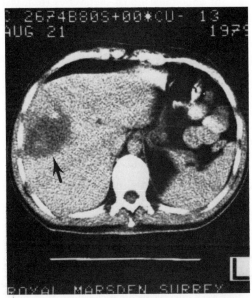

Fig. 19.7B CT scan through the liver in the same patient taken three weeks after therapeutic embolisation. This scan was also taken after intravenous contrast medium and shows a significant change in the attenuation values of the metastasis in the right lobe (arrowed) compared to the initial examination.

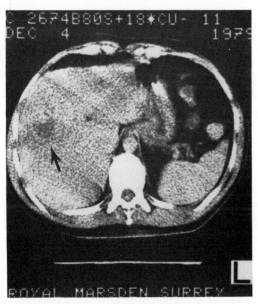

Fig. 19.7C CT scan of the same patient. Three weeks before this scan was taken the patient's symptoms of severe diarrhoea returned. The scan shows that the metastasis in the right lobe of the liver is more difficult to identify (arrowed) and the appearances are similar to the initial examination. This suggests that there has been tumour regrowth.

184

The results of CT volume changes and CT number changes in 6 patients treated with chemotherapy for abdominal nodal metastases from testicular teratoma, are shown in Figures 19.8A and B. The observations were made before each course of

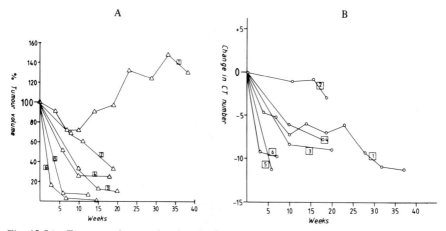

Fig. 19.8A   Tumour volume estimations in 6 patients with abdominal nodal metastases from testicular teratoma who were treated with chemotherapy. Observations were made on each patient at three to four week intervals before each course of chemotherapy. Tumour volume is shown on the ordinate and is expressed as a percentage of the initial absolute volume.
Fig. 19.8B   CT number estimations in the same patient as shown in Fig. 19.8A. CT number estimations are expressed on the ordinate as the change in CT number observed. Each reading represents the mean of multiple samples (each sample represented the mean attenuation value of 308 pixels). The standard deviations have not been shown in this figure for clearer representation.

chemotherapy. Tumour volume estimations show significant regression in 5 out of the 6 patients but in one patient initial regression was followed by a significant increase in tumour volume. CT number estimations show a progressive reduction in all patients. Thus, in 5 out of the 6 patients a similar pattern of decreasing tumour volume and decreasing CT number is seen. The diminishing attenuation values in response to treatment may reflect cystic degeneration which is known to occur in testicular teratomas. The significance of the results in the single patient in whom the tumour volume increased but the CT number decreased are speculative, but the finding may indicate that increase in size of a tumour does not necessarily represent tumour growth. At the Royal Marsden Hospital abdominal nodal resection is undertaken in selected patients following chemotherapy and radiotherapy (Hendry et al, 1980) providing the opportunity to study the relationship between tumour volume, CT number changes and histopathology.

Studies of tumour volume and CT number estimations have been extended to the investigation of pancreatic carcinoma. This tumour is much more difficult to delineate than retroperitoneal nodal masses because the attenuation values of the neoplasm are similar to normal pancreatic tissue (Sheedy et al, 1977). However, in selected patients the mass can be outlined (Fig. 19.9) but the errors incurred are likely to be higher than in patients with testicular teratoma. The preliminary results in patients with pancreatic carcinoma suggest that as in patients with

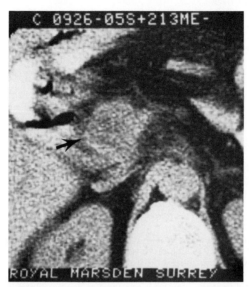

Fig. 19.9 CT scan of a patient showing a carcinoma in the head of the pancreas (arrowed). This tumour is clearly defined and tumour volume estimation is therefore feasible.

abdominal nodal metastases from testicular teratomas, there may be a correlation between changes in tumour volume and CT number. However, in pancreatic carcinomas the changes are less marked and an increase in tumour volume and CT number is seen more frequently than a decrease, probably reflecting the inadequacy of current therapy. These results are only preliminary and are therefore not discussed in detail in this paper but will be the subject of a further communication.

Conclusions

In this review an attempt has been made to illustrate the role of CT as a method of monitoring therapeutic response of tumours in the chest and abdomen. In the majority of patients such evaluation is subjective but the technique also permits quantitative studies of changes in tumour volume and tissue characteristics. These studies have important implications for examining the efficacy of different treatment regimes and for the study of tumour biology.

Acknowledgements

We are most grateful to Professor Peckham for allowing us to study patients under his care and for his continued encouragement and advice. We are indebted to Dr J.S. Macdonald and Dr Roy Parker for their support in carrying out this project. We gratefully acknowledge the Cancer Research Campaign and the Department of Health and Social Security whose generosity has made this work possible. Finally, we would like to thank Mrs Dorothy Mears for scanning the patients and Mrs Janice O'Donnell for typing the manuscript.

References

Breur K 1965 Growth rate and radiosensitivity of human tumours. Thesis University of Leiden. Mouton & Co., Den Haag

Collins V P, Loeffler R K, Tivey H 1956 Observation on growth rates of human tumours. American Journal of Roentgenology 76: 988-1000

Haefliger J M, Peckham M J, Steel G G 1979 Changes in lymph node size following systemic irradiation for the malignant lymphoma. Clinical Radiology 30: 5-10

Hendry W F, Barrett A, McElwain T J, Wallace D M, Peckham M J The role of surgery in the combined management of metastases from malignant teratomas of testis. British Journal of Urology 52: 38-44

Husband J E, Cassell K J, Peckham M J, Macdonald J S 1980 The role of computed tomography in the assessment of tumour volume in patients with malignant testicular teratoma. Presented at the European Association of Radiology Workshop on Computerised Tomographic Scanners in Radiotherapy in Europe. Geneva March 1979. British Journal of Radiology Special Report Series (in press)

Macdonald J S, Laugier A, Schlienger M 1968 Observations on the growth of tumours in lymph nodes changing from normal to abnormal while remaining opacified at lymphography. Clinical Radiology 19: 120-127

Sheedy P F, Stephens D H, Hattory R R, MacCarthy R L 1977 Computed tomography in the evaluation of patients with suspected carcinoma of the pancreas. Radiology 124: 731-737

Spratt J S, Spratt T L 1964 Rates of growth of pulmonary metastases and host survival. Annals of Surgery 159: 161

Steel G G, Lamerton L F 1966 The growth of human tumours. British Journal of Cancer 20: 74

Tyrrell C J, Peckham M J 1976 The response of lymph node metastases of testicular teratoma to radiation therapy. British Journal of Urology 48: 363-370

Welin S, Youker J, Soratt J S 1963 The rates and patterns of growth of 375 tumours of the large intestine and rectum, observed serially by double contrast enema study (Malmo technique). American Journal of Roentgenology 90: 673-686

20. The role of CT scanning in oncology

M. J. PECKHAM

During the past few years there have been major advances in imaging which have important implications for clinical oncology. In assessing this new technology it is important not to disregard proven methods for investigating tumours and information on the patterns of spread and relapse acquired by careful observation should be considered complementary to new developments in the field of imaging.

Since 1977 a multi-disciplinary team at the Royal Marsden Hospital, Sutton, has been engaged in a programme to evaluate the role of CT scanning in oncology. This programme has been conceived as a clinical research investigation and conducted through a series of protocols. Thus the facility was not generally available for routine clinical use within the hospital, so that the maximum information might be derived by directing efforts at a series of specific questions. The scope of the work included the following aspects:

A. Evaluation of the role of CT scanning in staging tumours at various sites
B. The role of CT scanning for monitoring tumour response to therapy and the early detection of recurrence and extension
C. Investigation of the role of CT scanning in radiation therapy planning.

A. Staging

However precise the tumour localisation method under consideration may be, very small aggregates of tumour will remain undetected and it is essential to interpret the findings in relation to the clinical behaviour of the tumour. For example, historical observation has shown that the majority of patients presenting with apparently localised Ewing's sarcoma of bone have disseminated subclinical metastases. In most patients these become clinically evident within the first year if treatment is confined to the primary tumour. An imaging technique applied to a clinical situation of this type may demonstrate metastases in a proportion of patients initially but a negative result would not signify the absence of metastatic disease.

CT scanning may contribute to staging in two ways: firstly, by detecting direct local extension from the primary tumour site more precisely and secondly, by detecting lymphatic and extralymphatic metastases. Two examples will be considered briefly.

1. Teratoma testis

Testicular teratoma shows an early propensity for spread to retroperitoneal, mediastinal and supraclavicular lymph nodes, the lungs and eventually the liver. In patients with Stage I disease (i.e. where following orchidectomy, conventional methods of clinical staging including lymphangiography and whole lung tomography fail to demonstrate evidence of metastatic disease), clinical experience has shown that this is a heterogeneous group comprising:

(a) patients who have no metastatic disease and who are cured by orchidectomy

(b) patients who have metastatic disease confined to the retroperitoneum

(c) patients in whom extension to the lung has already occurred but where conventional methods are incapable of demonstrating metastases

(d) patients where there is subclinical disease in the retroperitoneum and lungs.

Evidence for the curability by orchidectomy alone derives from historical experience before the advent of either radical node dissection or routine retroperitoneal node irradiation. Evidence for occult metastases in the retroperitoneum comes from data comparing histology of resected lymph nodes with lymphography which demonstrates that 25 per cent of patients with negative lymphograms have metastases in the lymph nodes. Evidence for occult metastases in the lungs derives from the study of spread patterns in Stage I patients treated with post-operative radiotherapy to the retroperitoneal nodes. In the latter group 20 per cent of patients relapse predominantly in the lungs and supradiaphragmatic lymph nodes (Peckham, 1979).

On the basis of this background experience, it was relevant to apply CT scanning to clinical Stage I patients to see whether the groups of patients indicated above could be defined more precisely. Table 20.1 shows the results obtained in a group

Table 20.1 Modified stage distribution of patients with clinical Stage I teratoma testis as a result of CT scanning (Husband J E, 1980)

Total Stage I patients pre-CT scan	% Stage distribution after CT scanning			
	I	II	III	IV
21	76.2	4.7		19

Stage I   :   No clinical evidence of disease after orchidectomy
Stage II :   Involved retroperitoneal lymph nodes
Stage III :   Supradiaphragmatic nodes
Stage IV :   Extralymphatic spread to lungs, etc.

of previously untreated patients and demonstrates that significant stage modification occurs due predominantly to the detection of lung metastases placing more patients in the Stage IV category. In addition, there is a smaller change in stage due to the detection of metastatic disease in the retroperitoneum in patients with negative lymphograms. These findings have important implications for management. Stage I patients who are shown to have pulmonary metastases receive intensive chemotherapy, whereas the Stage I patient who is CT scan negative may be managed by a policy of no treatment and careful observation following removal of the primary tumour, provided serum marker levels are persistently normal, or revert rapidly to normal, after orchidectomy. In pursuing a policy of this kind considerable reliance is placed upon the tumour imaging technique which raises the important issue of validating CT findings. It is essential that here and in other clinical situations CT findings need to be tested wherever practicable against direct observation and histological confirmation of the presence of tumour. This is not possible in every case since it would be unjustifiable to explore the lungs routinely in order to confirm the presence of lung metastases. However, it is important to test the validity of the CT prediction wherever practicable. Experience will be slow to accumulate but to date results indicate an encouraging degree of concordance.

2. Carcinoma of the bladder

In carcinoma of the bladder the intention was to see whether the extent of the primary lesion could be defined more accurately by CT and whether lymph nodes in the internal iliac region, normally not opacified at lymphography, could be demonstrated.

The results with respect to the lymph node findings were disappointing (Hodson et al, 1979) whereas the detection of the extent of the primary tumour yielded valuable information with significant stage changes as summarised in Table 20.2.

Table 20.2 Modification of stage of primary bladder carcinoma by CT scanning (Data from Husband & Hodson, 1980)

Stage prior to CT scan	No. of patients	% Distribution by T stage after CT scanning				
		T_2	T_{3a}	T_{3b}	T_{4a}	T_{4b}
T_2	14	28.6	50	21.4	–	–
T_3	36	–	27.8	63.9	8.3	–
T_{4a}	12	–	–	75	25	–
T_{4b}	13	–	–	46.2	–	53.8

Management by preoperative irradiation and surgery provides an opportunity to compare the surgical pathology of the resected tumour with the preoperative CT scan. Data on 14 patients summarised in Table 20.3 shows that, as expected, microscopic residua cannot be detected by CT. Extension into adjacent organs or into paravesical soft tissues in some instances has been deficient in this small experience, but more information is needed to allow more rigorous assessment of CT performance.

Table 20.3 Comparison of CT based clinical staging with surgical pathology in bladder carcinoma (Data from Husband & Hodson, 1980)

CT findings preoperatively	Thickened bladder wall – 5 patients	T_{3a} 2 patients	T_{3b} 6 patients	T_{4a} 1 patient
Pathological findings at surgery	2 microscopic tumour 3 negative	1–3b 1–4a	1–Histologically negative 2–3a 3–3b	1–4a

Improved staging in relation to clinical objectives

The potential role of CT and the applications which may be envisaged in various tumour sites are summarised in Table 20.4. One result of stage modification is the avoidance of radical therapy, e.g. the demonstration of haematogeneous spread may influence the decision whether or not to perform radical surgery in a patient with a bone or soft tissue sarcoma. In other clinical situations where more than

Table 20.4 CT findings with therapeutic implications

Tumour detected by CT scan	Tumour type
Pulmonary metastases	Teratoma testis Soft tissue, bone sarcomas
Abdominal node metastases	Pelvic carcinomas Lymphomas Teratoma testis
Contiguous extension	Head and neck carcinoma Carcinoma bladder
Tumour volume	Teratoma (Pancreas)

one treatment option is available (as indicated above for testicular teratoma), improved staging information allows for more selective deployment of different treatment options.

It is important that the overall clinical objective is clearly defined when CT is introduced into a staging protocol. In Hodgkin's disease, for example, the role of staging laparotomy is primarily to detect involvement of the spleen and it seems unlikely that CT will prove to be a satisfactory alternative to surgery in this respect. Equally pertinent to the role of CT in lymphoma, is the present uncertainty as to whether laparotomy or improved abdominal staging contributes to treatment results.

B. The role of CT for monitoring tumour response to therapy and the early detection of recurrence and extension

CT is a valuable method for following tumours on therapy, monitoring volume regression and detecting recurrence. Metastases in the lungs and retroperitoneum are particularly amenable to CT assessment. The development of a technique for calculating tumour volume by integrating surface areas from sequential CT sections is discussed in Chapter 19. In testicular teratomas the rate and extent of tumour regression is being investigated in relation to the rate of fall of serum markers to determine whether early change is predictive of eventual treatment outcome. Changes in tissue density within the tumour mass are being examined in relation to histology in an attempt to identify patients who have residual viable tumour.

Because of the influence of tumour volume on therapeutic sensitivity both for radiotherapy and chemotherapy, the early detection of relapse is of considerable clinical importance.

C. CT scanning in radiation therapy planning

An initial assessment of the role of CT in radiation therapy has been carried out, comparing plans derived using conventional methods of investigation and employing orthogonal simulator films with plans derived incorporating CT information. This has demonstrated significant deficiencies in the former method as summarised in Table 20.5 (Hobday et al, 1979). In some tumours, particularly pelvic tumours

Table 20.5 Impact of CT based planning in radiotherapy: Modification in treatment volume (Royal Marsden Hospital 1977–1980–Hodson N.J. unpublished data)

Primary tumour site	No. of patients	Treatment volume change	%
Intrathoracic	94	27	29
Head and neck	28	5	18
Retroperitoneum (including pancreas)	38	20	53
Pelvis	129	23	18
Total	289	75	25.9

and tumours of the head and neck, demonstration of stage change or change in extent of the primary tumour mass has not led to major modifcation in radiation therapy planning. This is because the fields generally employed include a margin so that possible sites of local extension are irradiated. In other sites, such as the lung and retroperitoneum, major changes have been demonstrated because of inadequate information on the localisation of tumour provided by previously available methods. Furthermore, accurate information on the disposition of normal structures has resulted in some patients, in a reduction in radiation dose to normal structures, such as the kidney. This information has increased flexibility in planning approach, for example, using three field techniques to irradiate the retroperitoneum. It is essential that radiation therapy planning is not based solely upon the CT image. Information on tumour spread and patterns of relapse following radiotherapy need to be retained and incorporated into the planning approach. The levels of detection which may be expected from clinical and pathological staging procedures and from an analysis of relapse patterns, are summarised in Table 20.6. As indicated it may be appropriate to consider CT information as a satisfactory basis for a Phase II or Phase III plan in which reduced and individualised treatment volumes are used to boost the tumour to a higher dose. The Phase I plan would include the tumour as demonstrated by CT as well as tissue where there is a high probability of local extension.

So far as the critical testing of the role of CT in radiation therapy planning is concerned the logical next step would be to examine the impact of improved imaging on therapeutic results. However, such a study poses problems. It is difficult to justify a randomised clinical study when it has been demonstrated that a proportion of patients planned for radical and potentially curative therapy without the benefit of CT, may not have the tumour completely included within the irradiated volume. As an alternative approach, patients having wide-field irradi-

Table 20.6 Expected levels of tumour detection from clinical and surgical staging procedures and clinical observation, in relation to radiotherapeutic approach

Tumour	Conventional clinical staging	Surgical staging	CT scan	Clinical analysis of relapse patterns following radiotherapy	Scope of Radiotherapeutic Approach		
					Phase I*	Phase II	Phase III
Primary tumour	+	+	+		+	+	+
Macroscopic loco-regional extension/metastasis	+	+	±		+	+	
Microscopic loco-regional spread	−	+	−	+	+		

*Phase I, II, III indicate progressive reduction in irradiated volume as therapy proceeds

ation, where the percentage changes in plans is low (for example, for bladder carcinoma), might be randomised between a traditional planning procedure and a plan which includes a Phase II based on CT information and used to deliver a boost dose to the tumour mass. The overall objective of CT in radiotherapy is summarised in Table 20.7.

Table 20.7 Rationale of CT scanning in radiation therapy

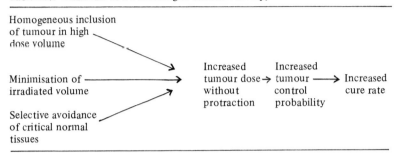

Radiation therapy planning in patients with chemosensitive tumours

A further and potentially valuable role for more precise radiotherapy planning is in patients with chemosensitive tumours where there is a high probability of eradicating small metastases but where failure with chemotherapy is related to the presence of bulky disease. In situations where the bulky disease requires radiotherapy it is important to minimise the amount of normal tissue included in the treatment volume because of the risk of enhanced normal tissue toxicity associated with combined therapy. In patients with bulky retroperitoneal lymph node metastases from teratoma testis, the extent of residual disease is identified by abdominal CT, following intensive chemotherapy, and a radiotherapy plan is then based on the scan information. In patients with Hodgkin's disease who have extensive mediastinal adenopathy, chemotherapy followed by radiotherapy is the treatment of choice; the precise delineation of mediastinal disease and the anatomical relationship of the heart to involved lymph nodes, which is difficult to define by conventional radiology, may be resolved by CT scanning.

Conclusions

It is clear that CT has a valuable role in clinical oncology. This role includes staging, monitoring of treatment response, detection of early relapse and radiation therapy planning. In addition, CT information may be useful for defining the most suitable surgical approach. The use of CT to obtain information on regression rates of human tumours is of biological interest and changes in tissue density within the tumour area may well become valuable for assessing response in those tumours where considerable tumour destruction is produced by treatment but where little reduction in volume may be observed.

It is important to identify clinical areas where CT is superficially attractive but where no obvious precise clinical objective can be defined. At the present time it is not clear that CT has a useful clinical role to play in the management of lymphomas.

Finally, it needs to be stressed that wherever possible CT information requires to be verified by histology since major modifications of treatment approach may depend upon the findings of this and other methods of tumour imaging.

References

Hobday P, Hodson N, Husband J, Parker K, Macdonald J 1979 Computed tomography applied to radiotherapy treatment planning: techniques and results. Radiology 133 (2): 477-482
Husband J E, Hodson N J 1980 Computerised axial tomography for staging and assessing response to treatment. In: Hendry W F, Oliver R T D, Bloom H J G (ed) Bladder cancer — principles of combination therapy. Butterworths, London (in press)
Husband J E 1980 The role of computed tomography in testicular teratomas. In: Peckham M J (ed) The management of testicular tumours. Arnold, London (in press)
Peckham M J 1979 An appraisal of the role radiation therapy in the management of non seminomatous germ-cell tumours of the testis in the era of effective chemotherapy. Cancer Treatment Reports 63: 1653-1658

Index